A SURVIVOR'S COOKBOOK

Guide to Kicking Hypothyroidism's Booty

A.L. CHILDERS

PAGE PUBLISHING, INC.
New York, NY

First originally published by Page Publishing, Inc. 2016

ISBN 978-1-68289-368-5 (pbk)
ISBN 978-1-68289-369-2 (digital)

Printed in the United States of America

A delicious gluten-free, grain-free, dairy-free, unprocessed, super-charge-your-metabolism, refuel-your-body, revitalize-thyroid-function, and shed-those-excess-pounds book! Along with bonus extras recipes for nontoxic house cleaning ideas. Over two hundred *easy* and *delicious* recipes for optimal thyroid nutritional well-being.

It's not about being skinny, it's about energy, vitality, and feeling good when you look in the mirror.

For delicious make-ahead meals, nothing beats a crock pot and they can be lifesavers for us busy cooks. There's nothing like the aroma of a home-cooked dinner welcoming you at the door.

Look for my second-edition book, *A Survivor's Cookbook: Guide to Kicking Hypothyroidisms Booty, The Slow-Cooker Way*

I've added a few bonus crock pot recipes to this collection is deliciously good-for-your thyroid recipes that are simple, delicious, and naturally gluten-free meals.

MESSAGE FROM THE AUTHOR

A personal favorite quote of mine is "From stressed to blessed." I mean this, believe, and receive this. I've been battling hypothyroidism for years, and I wanted to create a user-friendly handbook to help anyone affected by this disorder. I've seen many doctors over the years and none offered me ideas on diet change. I've included recipes, ideas on solutions for a healthier home, what you should be eating and shouldn't, how to shed those extra pounds, regain your self-confidence and vitality back into your life. I want you to feel strong, sexy, and beautiful. This is my heartfelt guide to you. Together, once again, you can start to gain that wonderful life that you deserve. I am a student in this thing called *life*. I want to be remembered as a pioneer who thought, imagined, and inspired. What we feel at times is the impossible or unthinkable. Life is a wonderful journey. Laugh at yourself as much as possible! Never try to walk someone else's path. You are destined for your own path and journey. I can't be you, and you can't be me. It's up to you to accept your journey and walk your path in life. Let's kick hypothyroidism's booty together!

DISCLAIMER

The information and recipes contained in this book are based upon the research and the personal experiences of the author. They are not intended as replacements for what your health care provider has suggested. The publisher and author are not responsible for any adverse effects or consequences resulting from the use of any of the suggestions, preparations, or procedures discussed in this book. All matters pertaining to your health should be supervised by a health care professional. I am not a doctor or a medical professional. This book is designed as an educational tool only. Please ask your health practitioner before taking any vitamins, supplements, or herbs, as they may have side effects, especially when combined with medications, alcohol, or other vitamins or supplements. Knowledge is power; educate yourself and find the answer to your health care needs. Wisdom is a wonderful thing to seek. I hope this book will teach and encourage you to take leaps in your life to educate yourself for a happier and healthier life. You have to take ownership of your health. Bottom line is you've got to be your own advocate for your health.

> Let food be thy medicine and medicine be thy food.
>
> —Hippocrates

ACKNOWLEDGEMENTS

I would like to thank everyone who has been curious and sought after the truth. All of us who were laughed upon, who stepped out of their comfort zone to make a difference not only in their health but the health and well-being of others. Most importantly, I would like to thank my husband, who has loved me at my craziest, encouraged me at my weakest, and have been a wonderful, loving, and kind father to our beautiful three daughters, Katlyn, Abbigail, and Caroline.

Let's feed your inner foodie!

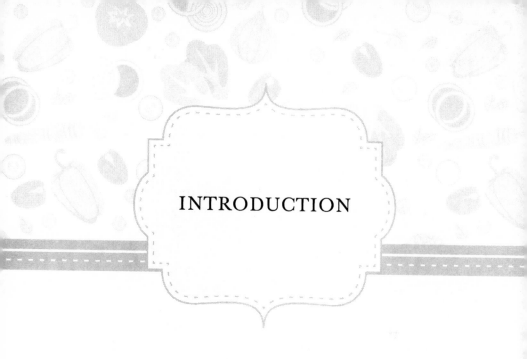

INTRODUCTION

Every disease has a starting point

We are one of the richest country in the world and we have an abundance of food everywhere it seems, but yet we are extremely malnourished and mineral deficient. *Why is that?* We are literally starving our bodies to death. *How can this be?* Our problem is that even with all of this abundance of food, readily available at our hands, people aren't obtaining the *basic nutrients* their bodies need in *order to fuel* what is needed to perform the necessary basic functions. The standard American diet in a nutshell is fatty, unbalanced, oversized, and loaded with cholesterol, salt, sugar, artificial ingredients, and preservatives. Sometimes if you look at things at a different angle, you grasp the *bigger picture* better. Think of your body as a car engine. A car's engine needs the right fuel, good lubricants, the engine serviced and tuned regularly. You want to make sure it runs smoothly and efficiently, reducing the risk of breakdowns. *Regular maintenance* of the engine is preformed to ensure its performance, reliability, and longevity! *Our heart is the pump of our human engine!* The heart pumps blood throughout your body. This blood provides your body with the oxygen and nutrients it needs. It also carries away waste. So, like a car, we need the *right fuel, which is food*; the right lubricants, which is the right fats—our engine, meaning a regular yearly checkup with bloodwork done and tuned regularly, meaning exercise. Just like a car's engine, everything in it is connected has a task. Our bodies are always trying to attempt to repair and heal itself.

Have you ever stopped to think what the underlying reason why you have hypothyroidism?

Many different underlying reasons can play a role. We do know that hypothyroidism is a chronic condition of an underactive thyroid and affects millions of Americans. Environmental chemicals and toxins, pesticides, BPA, thyroid endocrine disruptors, iodine imbalance, other medications, fluoride, overuse of soy products, cigarette smoking, and gluten intolerance. All of these play a very important role in your thyroid health. A nonprofit group called *Beyond Pesticides* warns that some 60 percent of pesticides used today have been shown to affect the thyroid gland's production of T3 and T4 hormones. Commercially available insecticides and fungicides have also been involved. Even dental x-rays have been linked to an increased risk of thyroid disorders.

Hypothyroidism means what exactly?

Hypothyroidism means your thyroid is not making enough thyroid hormone. Your thyroid is a butterfly-shaped gland in the front of your throat. It makes the hormones that control the way your body uses energy. Basically, our thyroid hormone tells all the cells in our bodies how busy they should be. Our bodies will go into overdrive with too much thyroid hormone (hyp*er*thyroidism) and our bodies slow down with too little thyroid hormone (hyp*o*thyroidism). The most common causes of hypothyroidism *worldwide is dietary and environmental.*

Hypothyroidism can cause many different symptoms:

Dry skin and brittle nails
Your fingertips becoming numb
Feeling fatigued, weak, or depressed

Constipation

Memory problems or having trouble thinking clearly

Heavy or irregular menstrual periods

Joint or muscle pain

Unexplained weight gain

Thinning hair

Clammy palms

Difficulty swallowing

Sensation of lump in throat

Dry, itchy scalp

Diminished sex drive

Persistent cold sores, boils, or breakouts

Elevated levels of LDL (the "bad" cholesterol) and heightened risk of heart disease

Heart Palpitations

Inability to lose weight

Inability to eat in the mornings

Tightness in throat; sore throat

Per The university of Marlyland Medical website http://umm.edu/health/medical/altmed/supplement/tyrosine. Tyrosine is a nonessential amino acid the body makes from another amino acid called phenylalanine. It is a building block for several important brain chemicals called neurotransmitters, including epinephrine, norepinephrine, and dopamine. Neurotransmitters help nerve cells communicate and influence mood. Tyrosine also helps produce melanin, the pigment responsible for hair and skin color. It helps in the function of organs responsible for making and regulating hormones, including the adrenal, thyroid, and pituitary glands. It is involved in the structure of almost every protein in the body.

Our bodies need tyrosine (an amino acid from dietary protein) and iodine (a naturally occurring salt) to make our thyroid hormone.

Here is a list of sample foods that are high in tyrosine:

Avocado (49 mg per ½ avocado)

Banana, medium-size (11 mg)

White beans and lentils (490 mg per cup)

Egg whites (151 mg each)

Fish (approx. 740 mg per 100 g)

Chicken breast (1,047 mg per 100 g)

Turkey (1,188 mg per 100 g)

Shrimp, 4 large (153 mg)

Gluten-free oats, cooked in water (320 mg per cup)
Pumpkin seeds (383 mg per oz)
Sesame seeds (208 mg per oz)

Hair, skin, and muscle mainly comes from our "dietary protein" intake. In fact, being protein-deficient can lead to fatigue, muscle weakness, hair loss, constant cravings, insomnia, muscle and joint pain, low energy, stress, a foggy brain, and many more other health issues. We've been taught that man has historically been carnivorous eaters, but that's not entirely true. Anthropologists have spent decades researching and studying our ancestors' diets. Anthropologists have discovered that our ancestors got most of their nutrition from collecting fruits and nuts. The meat from big mammals was a treat more than an everyday reality. Don't misunderstand what I am saying—we need protein; it is essential to our existence. Now, when you read "dietary protein," don't think I am referring to solely animal meat. *Per wedmd.com, an average adult is encouraged to get 10 percent to 35 percent of their day's calories from protein foods. That's about 46 grams of protein for women, and 56 grams of protein for men.* Here are sixteen examples resources for the nonmeat protein approach.

Quinoa (8 g per cup)
Chia (4 grams per 2 tablespoons)
Cooked spinach (5 grams per one cup). Limit your cooked spinach intake to twice per week. It's a Cruciferous vegetable and we shall get into that later in the book.
Cooked broccoli (4 grams per 1 cup serving). Limit your cooked spinach intake to twice per week. It's a cruciferous vegetable and we shall get into that later in the book.
Nuts (5 to 7 grams per 1/4 cup serving)
Eggs (6 grams per egg)
Chickpeas (6 grams per half cup serving)
Lentils (18 grams per 1 cup serving)
Beans (15 grams per 1 cup serving)
Hempseed (10 grams per 2 tablespoons)
Avocados (4 grams per fruit—yes, avocado is a fruit!)
Brown rice (5 grams per 1 cup serving)

Oatmeal (6 grams per 1 cup serving) . Try one of my many overnight oats recipes in the breakfast chapter.

Unsalted sunflower seeds (6 grams per 1/4 cup serving)

Raw almonds (4 grams per 2 tablespoon serving)

IODINE

Another thing many hypothyroid sufferers deal with is the lack of iodine in their body. Iodine is a critical essential trace element in our diet. Our bodies can't make iodine; therefore we have to rely on food to obtain it. This essential trace element is an absolute necessity for normal growth and development. In the year 1924, the Morton Salt Company, at the request of the government, historically started to add iodine to their salt mixture (in the form of potassium iodide). Table salt that you buy out of the store is bad for you anyway. "Table salt" has a list of other hidden chemicals. These chemicals include everything from manufactured forms of sodium solo-co-aluminate, iodide, sodium bicarbonate, fluoride, anticaking agents, toxic amounts of potassium iodide, and aluminum derivatives. So, the next time you go to grab that saltshaker, think of all the other little things you could be getting along with it. I'm here to shout it out to you! *You don't have to rely solely on salt to get your iodine.* But if you insist on "salting" your foods, go a must healthier, more natural route—Himalayan sea salt or Celtic sea salt. The benefits of getting enough iodine is that your metabolism will be able to function more properly. We are on a sodium overload with all the processed foods. Read labels. Watch your sodium intake from prepackaged foods. Try to avoid prepackaged foods. Good rule of thumb: *if it came from a plant, eat it; if it was made in a plant, don't.* You have plenty of food options to pick from that are naturally high in iodine. They range from seafood to potatoes, and it's nice to be able to have a variety of different foods. Even better news: everything on this list, you can eat to help your thyroid become healthier. Our bodies need an average of *150 micrograms of iodine per day.* Here are seventeen examples of food choices that have naturally occurring iodine:

1 medium baked organic potato with skin,
  60 micrograms of iodine
Dried seaweed (1/4 ounce), 4,500 micrograms of iodine
Cod fish (3 ounces), 99 micrograms of iodine
Shrimp (3 ounces), 35 micrograms of iodine
Himalayan crystal salt (1/2 gram), 250 micrograms of iodine
Baked turkey breast (3 ounces), 34 micrograms of iodine
Dried prunes (5 prunes), 13 micrograms of iodine
Navy beans (1/2 cup), 32 micrograms of iodine
Fish sticks (2 fish sticks), 35 micrograms of iodine
Tuna in water (3 ounces), 17 micrograms of iodine
Boiled eggs (1 large egg), 12 micrograms of iodine
Plain yogurt (1 cup), 154 micrograms of iodine
Bananas (1 medium banana), 3 micrograms of iodine
Lobster (100 grams), 100 micrograms of iodine
Cheddar cheese (1 ounce), 12 micrograms of iodine
Cranberries (4 ounces), 400 micrograms of iodine
Green beans (1/2 cup), 3 micrograms of iodine

The Dietary Guidelines for Americans recommend limiting sodium to less than 2,300 mg a day—or 1,500 mg if you're age fifty-one or older or if you are black or if you have high blood pressure, diabetes, or chronic kidney disease. Read labels; it seems everything has sodium in it. Our bodies are on a sodium overload!

Pink Himalayan salt is naturally rich in iodine, so it doesn't need to be artificially added in. It also helps to create an electrolyte balance in your body, increases hydration, regulates water content both inside and outside of cells, balance pH (alkaline/acidity), and help to reduce acid reflux, prevents muscle cramping, aids in proper metabolism functioning, strengthen bones, lower blood pressure, help the intestines absorb nutrients, prevent goiters, improve circulation, dissolve and eliminate sediment to remove toxins. So, how much is 1,500 mg of salt? It is 3/4 of a teaspoon. Unbelievable!

Check this this out: Hypothyroid Sea Spray for Your Skin

I'm such a big fan of the mineral magnesium. We need magnesium for our heart, kidneys, and muscles to function properly. It helps our bodies produce energy. People with high levels of magnesium in their bodies don't develop diabetes. Being deficient in this mineral can make you have very little energy, anxiety, panic attacks, PMS, heart palpitations, diabetes, kidney stones, and many more other health-related issues. Here's a sea spray recipe that will nourish your skin.

Sea spray for your skin ingredients:

> 1 cup of chamomile tea
> 1 tablespoon Himalayan salt
> Pinch of Epsom salt
> 2 drops of lavender essential oil

Heat your chamomile tea up in the microwave. Next, mix your salt and Epsom salt to your warm tea and stir until salt is completely dissolved. Pour in your spray bottle then add the lavender oil. Put the sprayer on it and mix well. Spray in your skin or just apply with a cotton pad. It's a wonderful treat for your skin; use it as part of your daily skin care routine.

Sea Salt Spray for Hair

You've probably seen many over-the-counter sea salt sprays for your hair. Who doesn't love that natural beachside causal look? My hair is naturally hard to manage, dry, and frizzy with a little bit of wave here and some actual curl there. These store-bought products on the shelves are loaded with hormone-disrupting ingredients too. Why not make your own natural hair spray product with the health benefits too!

Sea Salt Spray ingredients

> 1.5 cups warm water
> 2 tablespoon sea salt
> 2 teaspoon Epsom salt
> 2 tablespoon organic coconut oil
> 2 tablespoon aloe vera gel
> 5 drops essential oil, optional

Heat your water to almost boiling. Place pot to a cold eye on the stove. Next, add the sea salt and Epsom salt and keep stirring until both are dissolved. After they are completely dissolved, add the organic coconut oil. Keep on stirring until the oil has completely melted. And lastly but not least, add the aloe vera gel. If you want to add essential oils for an extra scent, add 3–5 drops. Stir until all is mixed and pour into a spray bottle. Spray on wet or dry hair.

SUGARS

Sugar can be hidden in everything we eat that is processed and packaged by mankind. *Did you know?* According to the American Heart Association (AHA), the maximum amount of added sugars you should eat in a day are the following:

Men: 150 calories per day (37.5 grams or 9 teaspoons).
Women: 100 calories per day (25 grams or 6 teaspoons).

Read the back of your labels: 4 grams of sugar equals to 1 teaspoon of sugar. A 12-ounce can of Coca-Cola has 35 grams of sugar, which is equals to 8.75 teaspoons of sugar. Or if you want to find out how many calories are actual sugar, you can multiply 4 x the amount of sugar (39g = 156).

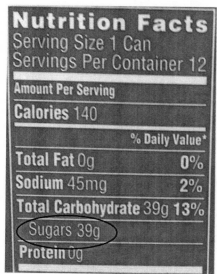

Standard Can of Soda

Let's do the calculation:

39g x 4 (4 calories/1g of sugar) = **156 calories**

This means there are **156 calories of sugar in every can of soda.**

* Note that there are more sugar calories than total calories noted on the label. This is allowable according to CFR-Code of Federal Regulations Title 21.

100% of the calories in every can is SUGAR!

Let's do a comparison of sugars hidden in foods. We all love a hot and now Krispy Kreme donut! That light comes on? I can eat three before I know it. It's so light and fluffy I can actually gobble them up before I even realize the donut has passed my lips. A Krispy Kreme donut has 10 grams of sugar in one donut. That equals out to 2.5 teaspoons of sugar per donut! Oh, and are they delicious!

Campbell's Classic Tomato Soup on the Go,
    20 grams (that's 5 teaspoons of sugar)
Dole Mixed Fruit Cup,
    17 grams (that's 3.5 teaspoons of sugar)
Prego Fresh Mushroom Italian Sauce,
    11 grams (that's 2.75 teaspoons of sugar)
Kraft French Style Fat Free Dressing,
    42 grams (that's 10.5 teaspoons of sugar)
All-natural Snapple Peach Tea,
    39 grams (that's 9.75 teaspoons of sugar)
Starbucks Caramel Frappuccino,
    64 grams (that's 16 teaspoons of sugar)
Quaker Instant Oatmeal, raisin, date, and walnut flavor,
    11 grams (that's 2.75 teaspoons of sugar)
Subway six-inch Meatball Marinara Sub,
    12 grams (that's 4 teaspoons of sugar)

KFC side of coleslaw,
    14 grams (that's 3.5 teaspoons of sugar)
Chobani Nonfat blueberry Greek yogurt,
    15 grams (that's 3.75 teaspoons of sugar)
Yoplait Original Yogurt Strawberry Banana,
    27 grams (that's 6.75 teaspoons of sugar)

We wonder why we can't lose weight—actually why we get fatter when we think we are trying to eat better by making better food choices. Low-fat, no fat, reduced, light—these are just some of the different names companies use to lure you in. STAY AWAY FROM THESE WORDS! If it walks like a duck and quacks like a duck, it *must* be a duck. Sugars can have many other names. Here are some other names for sugar, but it's still sugar!

THE 56 NAMES OF
SUGAR

Buttered syrup

Cane sugar

Brown sugar **Corn syrup** Cane juice Dextrose Caramel

Corn syrup solids

Beet sugar Confectioners' sugar Dehydrated cane juice Galactose

Agave nectar **Demerara sugar** Fruit juice concentrate

Fructose Maltodextrin **Diastatic malt** Diatase **Maltose**

Malt sugar Mannitol Florida crystals Molasses

Sucrose Sorghum syrup Sorbitol **Yellow sugar**

Carob syrup Treacle

Lactose **Panocha** Raw sugar **Rice syrup**

Castor sugar HFCS (High Frustose Corn Syrup) **Golden sugar** Muscovado

Barbados sugar **Glucose solids**

Barley malt Grape sugar Maple syrup Honey

Refiner's Syrup Sugar (granulated) **Turbinado sugar**

Golden syrup

Glucose Date sugar **Fruit juice** Icing sugar Dextran

Ethyl maltol

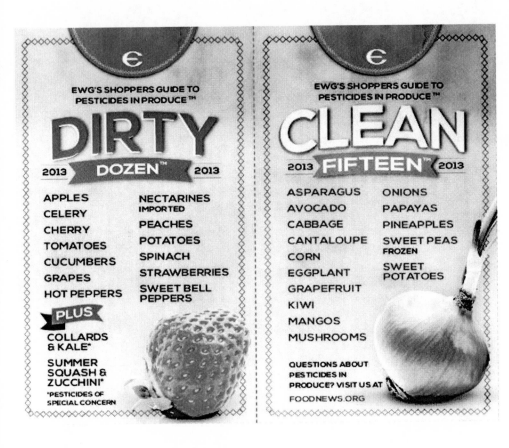

EWG'S SHOPPERS GUIDE TO
PESTICIDES IN PRODUCE ™

DIRTY

2013 DOZEN™ 2013

APPLES
CELERY
CHERRY
TOMATOES
CUCUMBERS
GRAPES
HOT PEPPERS

NECTARINES
IMPORTED
PEACHES
POTATOES
SPINACH
STRAWBERRIES
SWEET BELL
PEPPERS

PLUS

COLLARDS
& KALE*

SUMMER
SQUASH &
ZUCCHINI*

*PESTICIDES OF
SPECIAL CONCERN

EWG'S SHOPPERS GUIDE TO
PESTICIDES IN PRODUCE ™

CLEAN

2013 FIFTEEN™ 2013

ASPARAGUS
AVOCADO
CABBAGE
CANTALOUPE
CORN
EGGPLANT
GRAPEFRUIT
KIWI
MANGOS
MUSHROOMS

ONIONS
PAPAYAS
PINEAPPLES
SWEET PEAS
FROZEN
SWEET
POTATOES

QUESTIONS ABOUT
PESTICIDES IN
PRODUCE? VISIT US AT
FOODNEWS.ORG

EWG'S COMPLETE 2014 SHOPPER'S GUIDE TO PESTICIDES AND PRODUCE

(Other important findings in EWG's webpage)

- Every sample of imported nectarine were tested and 99 percent of apple samples tested positive for at least one pesticide residue.
- The average potato had more pesticides by weight than any other food.
- A single grape tested positive for 15 pesticides.
- Single samples of celery, cherry tomatoes, imported snap peas, and strawberries tested positive for 13 different pesticides apiece.
- Only 1 percent of avocado samples showed any detectable pesticides.
- There are 89 percent of pineapples, 82 percent of kiwi, 80 percent of papayas, 88 percent of mango, and 61 percent of cantaloupe that had no residues.

American Academy of Pediatrics issued an important report in 2012 that said that children have unique susceptibilities to pesticide residues' potential toxicity. By washing your food carefully, you protect the health of your whole family.

One of the biggest complaints I hear is, "I cant afford organic produce." That's okay. I have listed two recipes that can help try to minimize your pesticide exposure.

This natural vinegar wash is a good, cheap solution. Try this method of cleaning your produce even if you do buy organic. Some organic farmers use (natural) pesticides. Besides, you don't know who has actually touched the produce and if their hands where clean when handling it. Never hurts to take the extra precaution.

Recipes for washing your produce:

> Fill a bowl with water and add 1/2 cup of white vinegar, depending on the size of your bowl. (Basically its 3 parts water, 1 part vinegar)
> Place your fruits and veggies in the bowl.
> Soak for 15 to 20 minutes.
> Rinse with water.

Produce Spray

This all-natural pesticide-removing produce spray is really simple to make with ingredients you probably already have stored in your kitchen cabinets.

> 1 tablespoon lemon juice
> 2 tablespoons baking soda
> 1 cup water

Mix these ingredients until the baking soda has dissolved and pour into a clean spray bottle. Take a black permanent marker and write on your spray bottle, "Produce spray" and list the ingredients. (I always do this.) Spray the mixture onto your fruits and vegetables; sit the sprayed produce on a clean kitchen towel and let them sit for 10–15 minutes. After 15 minutes, rinse the mixture off and enjoy your produce!

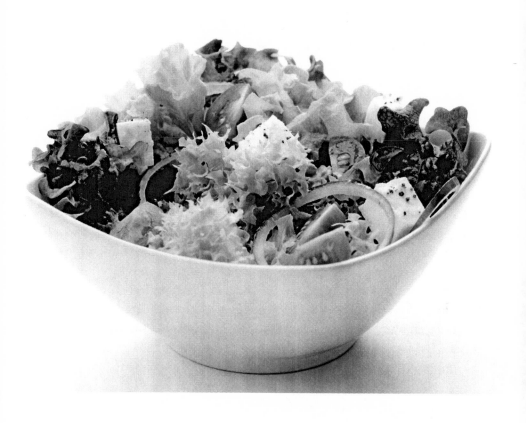

CRUCIFEROUS VEGETABLES

Cruciferous vegetables are a great source of fiber and are rich in nutrients, carotenoids, folate, antioxidants, minerals, and vitamins C, E, and K. There hasn't been any known human study that has demonstrated a deficiency in thyroid function from consuming *a limited amount of cooked* cruciferous vegetables. However, there has been a known case report to where an eighty-eight-year-old woman developed severe hypothyroidism and went into a coma after consuming an estimated 2–3 lbs of raw bok choy every day for several months. In fact, cruciferous vegetables protect against thyroid cancer and has many anticancer benefits. Cruciferous vegetables are rich sources of sulfur-containing compounds known as glucosinolates. Some glucosinolates found in raw cruciferous vegetables produces a compound known as goitrin, which has been found to interfere with thyroid hormone production. Very high intakes of raw cruciferous vegetables, such as raw cabbage and raw turnips, have been found to cause hypothyroidism. If someone developed hypothyroidism from consuming large amounts of cooked cruciferous vegetables. I would suggest that they have their iodine checked, and don't forget: everything in moderation. Limit your intake of cooked cancer-fighting veggies to a few times a week, but please eat your cancer-fighting veggies. The benefits clearly outweigh the risks.

Arugula
Bok choy, mustard greens
Broccoli Radish
Brussels sprouts, rutabaga
Cabbage, shepherd's purse
Cauliflower, turnip
Chinese cabbage, watercress
Collard greens
Daikon radish
Horseradish
Kale
Kohlrabi
Land cress

Diet does have a direct affect the way in which the body absorbs thyroid medication. You should always discuss with your doctor any dietary changes.

Tips

A diet for hypothyroidism should include whole foods rich in iodine: whole baked organic potatoes with skin, cod, dried seaweed, shrimp, Himalayan crystal salt, baked turkey breast, dried prunes, navy beans, tuna, boiled eggs, lobster, cranberries, and green beans. Niacin-rich foods (required for normal manufacture of thyroid hormone) are tuna, chicken, turkey, salmon, sardines, and brown rice. Riboflavin-rich foods are raw almonds, eggs, mushrooms, sesame seeds, salmon, and tuna. *Zinc (as well as vitamins B6, C, and E, iodine) is a major component of thyroid hormone balance and is antimicrobial.* Zinc-rich foods (boost thyroid function) are white cooked button mushrooms, chickpeas, kidney beans, dark chocolate (70 percent or higher), pumpkin, squash seeds, and almonds. Selenium-rich food (helps to convert T-4 to T-3) are Brazil nuts and tuna. High-polyphenols foods (acts as an anti-fungal) are cocoa powder, dark chocolate, coffee, tea, flaxseed meal, red raspberries, blueberries, black currants, Vitamin B6–rich foods (required for normal manufacture of thyroid hormone) are raw unsalted sunflower seeds, quinoa, raw pumpkin seeds, sesame seeds, flaxseeds, pistachio nuts, cashews, tuna, halibut, salmon, dried prunes, bananas, avocados, dried apricots, and raisins. Vitamin C–rich foods (boost thyroid gland function) are bell peppers, dark leafy greens, kiwis, broccoli, berries, citrus fruits, tomatoes, peas, and papayas. Riboflavin-rich foods (or vitamin b2—essential for normal manufacture of thyroid hormone) are frozen peas, beets, crimini mushrooms, eggs, asparagus, almonds, and turkey. Vitamin E–rich foods (work with zinc and vitamin A to produce thyroid hormone) are raw almonds, shrimp, avocados, quinoa, salmon, extra-virgin olive oil, and cooked butternut squash.

Eat foods that are rich in nutrients and minerals like veggies and fruits and make a choice to avoid artificial flavors, additives, and ingredients .

Take daily walks and meditation.

Take an Epsom salt baths three times per week or use the salt body spray recipe.

Remove parabens from all beauty products including makeup, shampoo, conditioner, soaps, sunscreen, dish soap, etc.

Try to get quality sleep 7–9 hours each night.

Never eat 3 hours prior to bedtime

Stop using chemically loaded dryer sheets. (I have a recipe in the back for a natural clothes softener)

Drink 1 tablespoon of Bragg's Organic Apple Cider Vinegar per day. (You can use Bragg's Organic Apple Cider Vinegar as a facial toner to fight acne and clear up skin.)

Use raw, organic, virgin, unfiltered coconut oil as a face and body moisturizer, hair conditioner; 1–3 tablespoon by mouth per day improves blood lipid, virgin coconut oil significantly reduced Total and LDL cholesterol, oxidized LDL, triglycerides, and increased HDL (the good) cholesterol help you lose weight and a dementia fighter.

Stay away from harsh household chemicals. Make you own cleaning supplies (recipes in back).

Take a daily probiotic. (At least three different strains and ten billion)

Stay away from nonstick cookware (contains toxic POAs and PFOAs that can break down your immune system). Avoid nonstick pans, pots, bakeware and utensils because they contain Teflon.

Use nonfluoride toothpaste! (Many brands out there that are non-fluoride or you can just simply use baking soda!)

Use aluminum-free deodorant (such as Tom's, other brands, or make your own, I have a recipe included).

Switch to purified water for both cooking and drinking to reduce fluoride consumption—fluoride has been implicated by some sources in reduced thyroid function. Black and green teas also contain fluoride.

Stay away from plastic bottles.

Did you know that most water bottles can contain phthalates, BPA and lead?

Bottled water is no safer than tap water. Did you know the FDA and EPA actually have stricter rules and guidelines for tap water than they do for bottled water? Yep, that's right!

Eat tyrosine-rich foods. Tyrosine is an amino acid that has an important role in the structure of almost all the protein found in your body. So eat more eggs, oats, tuna, salmon, lima beans, dulse flakes, almonds, pumpkin seeds, bananas, avocados and sesame seeds, chicken and turkey) Use cold-pressed olive oil and nuts for vitamin E, and nuts for some B vitamins. Eat nuts.

Two Brazil nuts per day will improve your selenium levels and give a boost to your immunity.

Start off with a glass of water and a broth-based soup or low-calorie, high-density salad.

Eat plenty of low-calorie, high-density foods: fruits, vegetables, gluten-free whole grains (quinoa, oats, brown rice, wild rice and corn) and beans

They don't pack a lot of calories per bite, but they fill you up because they are more water-rich and fiber-rich. You're basically getting more bang for your calorie buck!

Limit your intake of cruciferous vegetables, to twice a week and make sure they are cooked. Cruciferous vegetables can block the thyroid's ability to absorb iodine, which is essential for normal thyroid function. Please eat your cancer-fighting veggies. Here is a list of cruciferous vegetables:

Arugula
Bok choy
Broccoli

Brussels sprouts
Cabbage
Cauliflower
Chinese cabbage
Collard greens
Radish
Horseradish
Kale
Kohlrabi
Land cress
Mustard greens
Rutabaga
Turnip
Watercress

Avoid fermented or unfermented soy products like Tempeh, miso, tofu, and soy sauce

Try getting in a sauna or doing hot yoga to release heavy metals from your body.

Go sit in the sun for twenty minutes in the early morning hours per day and grab some free vitamin D. Let your arms, legs, and face be exposed (unless you take a medication where it states to avoid periods of sun exposure).

Nutritional deficiencies play a big role in thyroid dysfunction. These include deficiencies of iodine, vitamin D, omega-3 fats, selenium, zinc, vitamin A, and the B vitamins.

Gluten intolerance, food allergies, and heavy metals also place a role in hypothyroidism.

Exercise has been well established to decrease/eliminate risk of cancer, diabetes, heart disease, and even dementia while eating correctly. Every time you eat something, you need to think.

Make sure you see your doctor regularly and have your thyroid checked regularly. Have your doctor check all your levels.

Most importantly, stay away from negative people! People can add unwanted and unneeded stress.

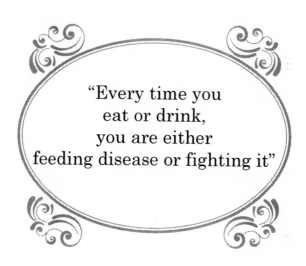

"Every time you
eat or drink,
you are either
feeding disease or fighting it"

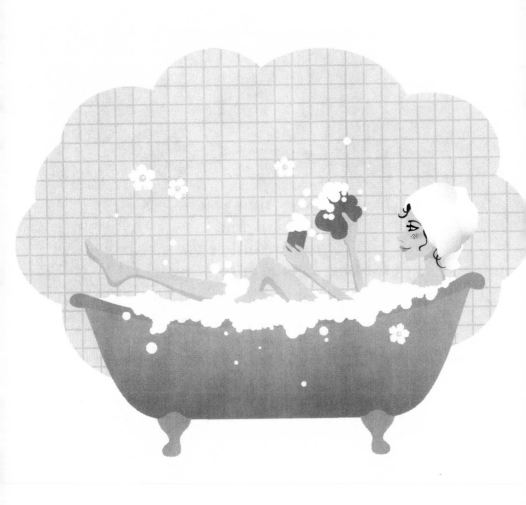

WHAT ARE THE BENEFITS TO MY HEALTH IF I WERE TO TAKE EPSOM BATHS?

Many of us are deficient in magnesium and we don't even know it. Magnesium is the second most abundant element in our cells, helps to regulate our bodies 325 enzymes, and plays an important role in organizing many bodily functions, like muscle control, electrical impulses, energy production, and the elimination of harmful toxins.

According to the National Academy of Sciences, American's magnesium deficiency helps to account for high rates of heart disease, stroke, osteoporosis, arthritis and joint pain, digestive maladies, stress-related illnesses, chronic fatigue and a number of other ailments.

Epsom salt is rich in magnesium and sulfate in which are easily absorbed through the skin. *Per* www.uhichicago.com *Sulfates help to form brain tissue, joint proteins and the proteins that line the walls of the digestive tract.* Sulfates also help detoxify the body of medicines and environmental contaminants.

The Epsom Salt Industry Council has listed many reasons why we should take an Epsom bath three times a week. Here are some other health benefits and eight different recipes for a relaxing, unwinding, and "wash the day off" detox bath. Be creative; find the scents that you like and mix your very special detox bath blends.

Improves heart and circulatory health, reducing irregular heart-
beats, preventing hardening of the arteries, reducing blood
clots and lowering your blood pressure.

Improves ability for the body to use insulin, reducing the inci-
dence or severity of diabetes.

Flushes toxins and heavy metals from the cells, easing muscle
pain, and helping the body to eliminate harmful substances.

Improves nerve function by electrolyte regulation. Also, calcium
is the main conductor for electrical current in the body, and
magnesium is necessary to maintain proper calcium levels in
the blood.

Relieves stress.

Reduces inflammation to relieve pain and muscle cramps.

Improves oxygen use.

Improves absorption of nutrients.

Prevents or eases of migraine headaches.

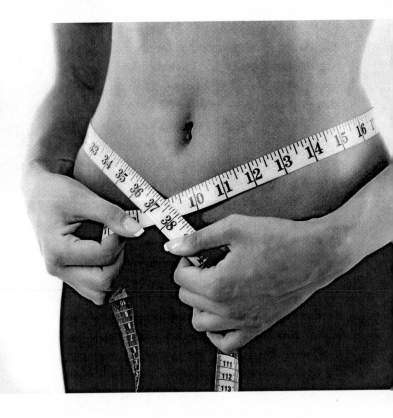

What is the slim and sassy essential oil blend? It's a blend of grapefruit, lemon, peppermint, ginger, and cinnamon. This metabolic blend can be used for weight loss, increased energy, increased metabolism, appetite suppression, and fighting those nasty, overwhelming cravings. You can purchase this essential oil pretty much anywhere or go to my blog website http://thehypothyroidismchick.com/ and follow me on twitter @thyroidismchick.

DIY Skin Smoother Detox Bath

2 cups Epsom salt
2 cups baking soda
2 cups sea salt
1 cup vinegar
1/4 cup of organic coconut oil (this will melt in the hot bath)

Combine the dry ingredients; store in a closed container. When you are ready to take a bath, add 1 cup of dry ingredients, 1 cup of vinegar, and 1/4 cup of coconut oil. (Kids can use up to a 1/2 cup of the mixture.) Bathe 3 times weekly, soaking for at least 12 minutes.

Soothing Lavender Detox Bath

2 cups Epsom salt
2 cups baking soda
5–10 drops of lavender oil

Combine the dry ingredients; store in a closed container. When you are ready to take a bath, add 1 cup of dry ingredients. (Kids can use up to 1/2 cup of the mixture.) Bathe 3 times weekly, soaking for at least 12 minutes.

Lavender Mint Bath

2 cups Epsom salt
2 cup baking soda
1 cup sea salt
10 drops of lavender essential oils
10 drops of peppermint essential oil

Combine the dry ingredients; store in a closed container. When you are ready to take a bath, add 1 cup of dry ingredients. (Kids can use up to 1/2 cup of the mixture.) Bathe 3 times weekly, soaking for at least 12 minutes.

Soothing Oatmeal Bath Salt Recipe

2 cups of Epsom salt
1 cup of sea salt
1.5 cups of finely pulverized oatmeal
10 drops of lavender essential oil

Grind the oatmeal finely in a food processor or spice grinder. You want it about the consistency of sugar or salt. Add the salts and lavender oil. Mix everything together well. Add 1 cup of the oatmeal-salt mixture under the running water and give a good stir. Store in a closed container. (Kids can use up to 1/2 cup of the mixture.) Bathe 3 times weekly, soaking for at least 12 minutes.

Goats Milk Bath

2 cups of powdered goat's milk
2 cup of Epsom salt
1 cup of sea salt
2 cup of baking soda
10 drops of lavender essential oil

Combine the dry ingredients and the lavender essential oil. Store in a closed container. When you are ready to take a bath, add 1 cup of dry ingredients. (Kids can use up to 1/2 cup of the mixture.) Bathe 3 times weekly, soaking for at least 12 minutes.

Basic bath salt

2 cups of Epsom salt
2 cups of sea salt
2 cups of baking soda

Combine the dry ingredients. Store in a closed container. When you are ready to take a bath, add 1 cup of dry ingredients. (Kids can use up to 1/2 cup of the mixture.)

Invigorating Foot Soak

    2 cups of Epsom salt
    2 cups of sea salt
    2 cup of baking soda
    10 drops of lavender essential oil
    5 drops of tea tree essential oil
    10 drops of peppermint essential oil

Combine the dry ingredients and the essential oils. Store in a closed container. When you are ready to use, put 1/2 cup of the mixture in your foot bathe. (Kids can use up to 1/2 cup of the mixture.)

After soaking your feet, be sure to dry them well; lather your feet with some coconut oil and place them in fresh clean socks.

Remember: always check with your doctor before starting this or any detox regimen. Especially if you are suffering from any sort of other health issues. Do not do a detox bath if you are pregnant, dehydrated, have heart problems, or have open sores (the salt will burn!).

Sugar Scrub for Dry skin

    1 cup brown sugar
    1/2 cup coconut oil
    1/4 cup raw honey
    2 teaspoon baking soda

Mix all your all ingredients in a mason jar and label Sugar Scrub on the container. Wet your sponge, but not dripping wet, and scoop out an adequate amount of the sugar scrub on it.

Exfoliate your skin gently using your bath sponge. Be careful not to scrub too hard. You want to scrub gently, just enough to remove the dead skin cells but not so it irritates your skin.

Rinse the mixture off in your shower. Pat dry your skin with your towel.

MORNING RISE
AND SHINE!

Most doctors recommend taking your thyroid medication in the morning before breakfast, on an empty stomach. Drink a full glass of freshly squeezed warm lemon water with your medication. (Take 1 lemon and squeeze into a 24 oz. glass of water. You can add a dash of cayenne for an extra kick.) Why drink warm lemon water with my thyroid medication, you ask. Warm lemon water serves as the perfect *good morning drink, pick-me-up drink,* as it aids the digestive system, being a rich source of nutrients like calcium, potassium, vitamin C and pectin fiber, calcium, phosphorus, and magnesium. It also plays the role of a blood purifier; has great antiseptic properties; helps reduce pain and inflammation in joints and knees as it dissolves uric acid; strengthens the liver by providing energy to the liver enzymes; helps replenish body salts especially after a hard, sweaty workout session; helps with body hydration, constipation; reduces phlegm; freshens breath; gives your immune system a boost; reduces inflammation; can help relieve or prevent digestive problems like bloating, intestinal gas, and heartburn; and lastly, weight loss. Cold water shocks your system and slows it down. Eat within the first hour of waking up. Do not take any other medications along with your thyroid. Avoid drinking juice, coffee, or anything other than water with your medication. Food and drinks will dilute the effectiveness, making your body absorb less than the prescribed amount. Your thyroid medication will help jump-start your metabolism and give you energy for the day. You can drink your coffee one hour after you've taken your medication. Several studies have shown that drinking coffee or espresso along with or shortly after taking thyroid tablet can significantly lower the absorption of the thyroid medication. If you absolutely have to coffee as your first initial am drink then speak with your doctor about taking your thyroid medication at night before bed. You also should wait four hours after taking your thyroid medication to take any calcium or iron supplements. It too can interfere with the absorption of your thyroid medication.

Change your toothpaste to a nonfluoride toothpaste brand. Fluoride is used as a drug to treat hyperthyroidism, an overactive thyroid, because it makes the thyroid underactive quite effectively. Change your water to filtered water or fluoride-free bottled water. A statement released January 2, 1997, from the EPA reads, "Indicates a causal link between fluoride/fluoridation and cancer, genetic damage, neurological impairment, and bone pathology."

Not everyone should avoid fluoride like the black plague, but we hypothyroid sufferers should minimize the consumption as much as possible. Don't forget to get your daily dose of sunlight. The sunlight stimulates the pineal gland, which in turn positively affects the thyroid as well as all the other endocrine glands. Some studies have found that between five and thirty minutes of sun exposure to your unprotected face, arms, legs or back between the hours of 10:00 a.m. and 3:00 p.m. two to three times every week is enough for your body to produce all the D3 it needs (source: National Institutes of Health - Office of Dietary Supplements).

Now, to the good stuff!

After reading all this, you may be thinking, *What exactly can I eat? How can I afford to eat better?* If you don't eat well now, you will pay later with your health. Your body will eventually start to break down. These recipes are designed to help you shed the weight and get your thyroid back into a working powerhouse! Everything in moderation. You have many different tasty recipes option to pick from this book to help you stay on track. *Healthy is the new skinny!* I am sharing my years of research with you to help empower, educate, and enlighten you on your journey to a healthier thyroid! All these recipes that I have gathered, collected, and developed are geared strictly to the well-being of our thyroid. Ideally you want to eat two servings of fruit and three servings of vegetables per day. Here are over 200 of my family's favorite recipes. I always say have Google will travel! Please research thyroid-friendly foods that you like and make your own family thyroid-friendly recipes.

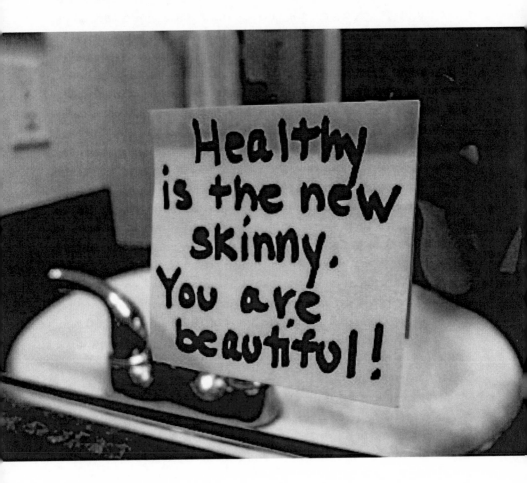

Foods you should concentrate more on eating with hypothyroidism:

Fatty fish like wild salmon, trout, halibut, cod, albacore tuna, flounder, cod or sardines (omega-3s and selenium) only a few times per week.... No farmed fish, period!

No gluten.

Split peas, lentils, black beans, kidney beans, pinto beans, artichokes, raspberries, blackberries, chia seeds, red apples with skin, prunes, green peas, raw almonds, garbanzo beans, winter squash, spaghetti squash, summer squash, butternut squash, zucchini, popcorn (no microwave-ready, bagged popcorn), cherries, citrus fruits, kiwi, cantaloupe, papaya, mango, plums and red grapes, tomatoes, carrots, gluten-free, steel-cut oats or gluten-free rolled oats, watermelon, green tea, organic apple cider vinegar, lemon, garlic, leeks, parsley, celery, ginger root, tomatoes, cucumbers, carrots, asparagus, organic whole baked potatoes with skin, shrimp, Himalayan crystal salt, Celtic sea salt, baked turkey breast, dried prunes, navy beans, gluten free steel cut or rolled oats, cranberries and green beans, organic no hormone-chicken, brown rice, raw almonds, eggs, sesame seeds,, chickpeas, kidney beans, dark chocolate 70 percent or higher, walnuts, cocoa powder, hempseeds, red raspberries, blueberries, black currants, brazil nuts, raw unsalted sunflower seeds, quinoa, raw pumpkin seeds, sesame seeds, flaxseeds, pistachio nuts, cashews, dried prunes, bananas, avocados, dried apricots, and raisins, red, green and orange bell peppers, romaine lettuce, kiwis, papayas, beets, all mushrooms, quinoa, extra-virgin olive oil and cooked butter nut squash. sea vegetables, dried seaweed (kelp, dulse, hijiki, nori, arame, wakame, kombu, tomato paste, brewer's yeast, brown rice, algae, healing spices (Ceylon cinnamon, turmeric, gloves, cayenne pepper, garlic, oregano, sage, ginger) .

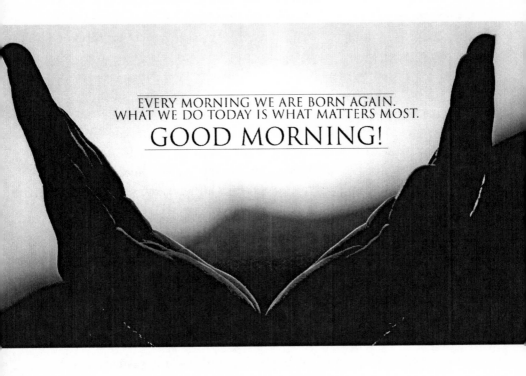

EVERY MORNING WE ARE BORN AGAIN.
WHAT WE DO TODAY IS WHAT MATTERS MOST.

GOOD MORNING!

Breakfast is the most important meal of the day. Never, ever skip breakfast. The right breakfast foods can help your concentration, give you energy, and get your metabolism moving to help you maintain a healthy weight. The aspiration to lose weight is one of the most frequently given for skipping breakfast. Many observational studies have found that people who skip breakfast are more likely to be overweight. *Your body thinks it starving so the natural self-preservation thing to do is to store fat. Your body will go into starvation mode and store fat!* Breakfast immediately raises the body's energy level and restores the blood glucose level to normal after a sleep-induced, overnight fast. Eating breakfast also lowers the blood level of the stress hormone cortisol. I know, with hypothyroidism, you're just not hungry in the morning. This is one of my side effects from having hypothyroidism.

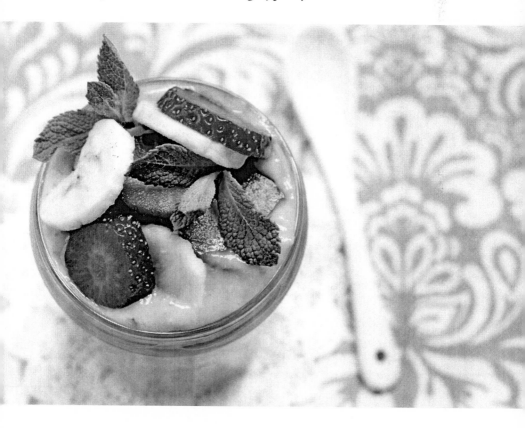

BREAKFAST
RECIPES

I want to teach you how to make perfect overnight oats in a jar and make your mornings totally effortless, quick, and not have a reason to *not eat breakfast*. The initial idea for making overnight oats is to make your mornings simpler and much more effortless. You need gluten-free, steel-cut (crunchy) oats or gluten-free rolled oats (smoother), a liquid component (yogurt, almond milk, or coconut milk, etc.), and some flavorings (fruit, spices, etc.). Add in extras like chia, hemp, or flaxseeds if you want a nutrition boost. Then let it all sit overnight while the oatmeal absorbs the liquid. I have given you a sample of recipes that my family enjoys, but be creative; use your own taste buds and make your very own versions of what you like.

The Basic Overnight Oats

> 1/3 cup GF steel-cut or rolled oats (steel-cut for a crunch or rolled oats for a smoother oatmeal)
> 1/3–1/2 cup almond milk or coconut milk (depending on how thick you like it)
> 1/3 cup plain So Delicious Greek-style yogurt
> 1/2 banana, mashed

1/2 tablespoon chia seeds (omega-3 fatty acids)
1/2 teaspoon ground cinnamon

Stir everything together in a bowl. Put in a mason jar with lid. Refrigerate for at least 6 hours, preferably overnight.

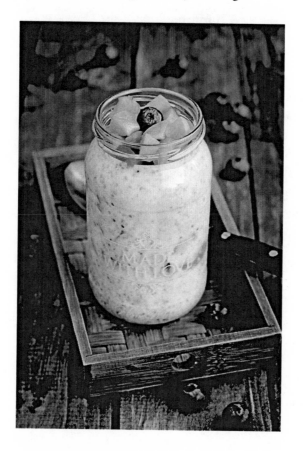

Overnight Chia Oatmeal with Fruit

1 tablespoon black chia seeds
1/4 cup oats
1/2 cup no sugar added vanilla almond milk
    (nut allergy: use coconut milk)
1 tablespoon ground flaxseeds or flaxseed meal
2 tablespoons dried apricots, minced in small edible pieces
1 teaspoon raw honey

Add all the ingredients to an 8-ounce mason jar. Cover with a lid and gently shake until the ingredients are combined.

Refrigerate for at least 6 hours, preferably overnight. When ready to eat, give the oats a good shake and dig in!

Almond Butter and Banana Overnight Oats

> 1 large ripe banana, mashed (about 1/2 cup)
> 1/4 cup creamy almond butter
> 1 cup GF steel cut or rolled oats (steel cut for a crunch or rolled oats for a smoother oatmeal)
> 1 cup unsweetened almond milk
> 1 tablespoon chia seeds (optional) (omega-3 fatty acids)
> 1/2 teaspoon vanilla extract
> 1/2 teaspoon ground cinnamon
> 1 teaspoon raw honey

In a medium bowl, mash your banana with a fork. Add the remaining ingredients to the bowl and mix until well combined. Pour the mixture into two 8-ounce mason jars with lids, seal tightly, and refrigerate for at least 6 hours, preferably overnight.

When ready to eat, give the oats a good shake and dig in!

Almond Butter Chocolate Overnight Oats

> 1/2 cup GF steel-cut or rolled oats (steel-cut for a crunch or rolled oats for a smoother oatmeal)
> 1 teaspoon chia seeds
> 1 teaspoon flax meal
> 2 teaspoon cacao powder
> 1 T almond butter
> 1 chopped Medjool date or 2 teaspoon grade B maple syrup
> 1/2 cup almond milk

Pour the mixture into an 8-ounce mason jars with lids, seal tightly, and refrigerate for at least 6 hours, preferably overnight. When ready to eat, give the oats a good shake and dig in!

Apple Cinnamon Overnight Oats

1/2 cup GF steel-cut or rolled oats (steel-cut for a crunch or rolled oats for a smoother oatmeal)
1 teaspoon chia seeds
1 teaspoon flax meal
1/2–1 teaspoon of cinnamon (depending on how strong you like it to be)
1/4 teaspoon vanilla extract
1/4 teaspoon nutmeg
1-2 T unsweetened applesauce
1–2 teaspoon grade B maple syrup (optional)
1/2–3/4 cup almond milk (depending on how thick or thin you like your oatmeal; nut allergy: use coconut milk)

Pour the mixture into an 8-ounce mason jars with lids, seal tightly, and refrigerate for at least 6 hours, preferably overnight. When ready to eat, give the oats a good shake and dig in!

Apricot Ginger Overnight Oats

1/4 cup GF steel-cut or rolled oats (steel-cut for a crunch or rolled oats for a smoother oatmeal)
1/2 cup almond or coconut milk
1/4 cup low-fat almond or coconut milk yogurt
1–1/2 teaspoons dried chia seeds (omega-3 fatty acids)
1 teaspoon raw honey, optional
   (or substitute any preferred sweetener)
1/8 teaspoon almond extract
3 dried apricots, diced (or 1/4 cup fresh)
1 teaspoon crystallized ginger, minced

In an 8-ounce mason jar, add oats, milk, yogurt, chia seeds, almond extract, and honey. Put lid on the mason jar and shake until well combined. Remove lid, add apricots and ginger, and shake again until well combined. Seal the jar with the lid and refrigerate for at least 6 hours, preferably overnight. When ready to eat, give the oats a good shake and dig in!

Banana Chocolate Overnight Oats

> 2 cups GF steel cut or rolled oats (steel cut for a crunch or rolled oats for a smoother oatmeal)
> 1 1/2 cups of almond or coconut milk
> 1/2 cups almond or coconut yogurt
> 1–2 tablespoon cocoa
> 1 tablespoon of ground flaxseed (omega-3 fatty acids)
> 1 tablespoon raw honey or grade B maple syrup

Pour the mixture into two 8-ounce mason jars with lids, seal tightly, and refrigerate for at least 6 hours, preferably overnight. When ready to eat, give the oats a good shake and dig in!

Blueberry Maple Overnight Oats

> 1/3 cup GF steel-cut or rolled oats (steel-cut for a crunch or rolled oats for a smoother oatmeal)
> 1/3 cup almond milk or coconut milk
> 1/4 cup almond or coconut milk Greek yogurt
> 1–1/2 teaspoons dried chia seeds (omega-3 fatty acids)
> 2 teaspoons grade B maple syrup (more or less to taste)
> 1/4 cup blueberries (or enough to fill jar)

Pour the mixture into an 8-ounce mason jar with lid, seal tightly, and refrigerate for at least 6 hours, preferably overnight. When ready to eat, give the oats a good shake and dig in!

Gingerbread Overnight Oats

> 1/2 cup GF steel-cut or rolled oats (steel-cut for a crunch or rolled oats for a smoother oatmeal)
> 1/2 cup almond milk (nut allergy: use coconut milk)
> 1 teaspoon chia seeds (omega-3 fatty acids)
> 1 teaspoon flax meal
> 1/2 teaspoon cinnamon
> 1/2 teaspoon ginger
> 1 teaspoon black strap molasses

2 teaspoons grade B maple syrup
1 teaspoon vanilla extract

Pour the mixture into an 8-ounce mason jar with lid, seal tightly, and refrigerate for at least 6 hours, preferably overnight. When ready to eat, give the oats a good shake and dig in!

Pumpkin Overnight Oats

1/2 cup GF steel-cut or rolled oats (steel-cut for a crunch or rolled
    oats for a smoother oatmeal)
1/4 teaspoon pumpkin pie spice
Pinch of fine sea salt
1/4 cup water
1/4 cup almond milk (nut allergy: use coconut milk)
3–4 tablespoons pumpkin puree
1/4 teaspoon black strap molasses
2 tablespoons grade B maple syrup
Raw pumpkin seeds

Mix everything together in a bowl. Pour the mixture into two 8-ounce mason jars with lids, seal tightly, and refrigerate for at least 6 hours, preferably overnight.

Pumpkin Quinoa Porridge

1 cup dry quinoa rinsed and drained
1 and 1/2 cups almond milk, divided
    (nut allergy: use coconut milk)
1/2 cup pumpkin puree
1 teaspoon cinnamon
1/2 teaspoon ginger
1/8 teaspoon cloves
1/8 teaspoon pink Himalayan sea salt
2 tablespoons ground flaxseeds
2–3 tablespoons raw honey or grade B maple syrup,
    more as desired

Bring 1 cup of the almond milk to a boil. Add the quinoa, pumpkin puree, cinnamon, ginger, cloves, and salt. Turn the heat down to a simmer and cook for 10 minutes or until the liquid has been completely absorbed.

Take off the heat and stir in the ground flaxseeds. Put your porridge in a bowl and add about 1/2 cup more of almond milk. Give it a good stir. To add an extra zing top your porridge with some sliced raw almonds or raw honey or grade B maple syrup and coconut flakes.

Chickpea, Tomato and Zucchini Frittata

Eggs are among one of the healthiest foods on the planet. Eggs are particularly rich in the two antioxidants lutein and zeaxanthin. Eggs are loaded with high-quality proteins, vitamins, minerals, good fats, and various trace nutrients; 6 grams of protein with all nine essential amino acids. Rich in iron, phosphorous, selenium, and vitamins A, B12, B2, and B5. Make sure to purchase omega-3-rich eggs, free roaming, and organic, not factory raised. Not all eggs are created equal. Stay away from your standard supermarket eggs. The chickens are usually raised in an overfilled henhouse or a cage and never see the light of day. They are usually fed a grain-based feed that are supplemented with vitamins and minerals, antibiotics, and hormones. So like the commercial states, it really is the incredible, edible egg!

    2 tablespoons vegetable or olive oil
    1 onion, thinly sliced
    1 zucchini, thinly sliced
    1/2 cup of cherry tomatoes, cut in half
    1 can (15 oz.) chickpeas, drained
    1 garlic clove, crushed
    1/2 teaspoon chili flakes
    1/2 teaspoon ground cumin
    3 tablespoon chopped flat-leaf parsley
    6 organic, cage-free eggs

Heat oil in a cast-iron skillet. Add onion and sauté over medium heat for 6–8 minutes or until golden brown. Add zucchini and tomatoes, increase the heat and sauté for 4 minutes or until softened. Stir in chickpeas, garlic, chili flakes, cumin and parsley and stir-fry for 2 minutes or until hot.

Beat eggs with 2 tablespoons water and stir into vegetables. Place in oven and cook on 350 degrees for about 20 minutes until its set.

Mushroom-Stuffed Omelet

Having mushrooms, onions, and eggs are a great way to boost selenium levels. Here is a quick recipe that is both filling and super easy to whip up.

    4 organic or cage-free eggs
    3 medium-sized mushrooms, diced
    1/2 tablespoon coconut oil or 1/2 tablespoon of avocado oil
    A teaspoon of dairy-free and soy-free butter
    Salt and pepper to taste

In a cast iron skillet, add 1/2 tablespoon of coconut oil or avocado oil and sauté the mushrooms till they are golden brown. While mushrooms are browning, whisk eggs with seasonings in a bowl. After the mushrooms have browned, add the teaspoon of butter. Stir the butter around the pan so it can get completely coated and mixed with the mushrooms.

Add the egg mixture. It will take about 1 minute for the egg to set and then flip over. Heat for another 30 seconds then remove from pan. Place on a plate.

Serve it with a piece of gluten-free toast, tomatoes, or some approved fruit.

Banana Brazil Nuts Pancakes

    1 large ripe banana
    1 teaspoon vanilla
    2 eggs, large
    3 tablespoon melted unsalted, organic, dairy-free butter (reserve
        1 tablespoon)
    1 1/2 cup goat's milk
    1/4 teaspoon salt

1/2 teaspoon baking soda
1 1/2 teaspoon baking powder
1 tablespoon raw honey
1 1/2 cups flour, gluten-free
4 Brazil nuts, grated
Grade B maple syrup

In a bowl, whisk together all the dry ingredients. In another bowl, whisk all the wet ingredients. Pour the wet ingredients into the flour mixture and mix. Mash the bananas in a bowl. Add the nuts and blend the mashed bananas into the batter. Use the reserved 1 tablespoon of butter and melt in the cast-iron skillet. Make sure the entire pan is coated to avoid sticking. Set your stove to medium heat. Cook the pancakes according to the size you want buy pouring batter in batches. Bubbles will start to appear on the surface. This tells you that they are ready to be flipped. Turn and cook an extra 2 minutes until it is brown and golden. Never hurts to experiment, and it makes it fun and less boring! Top with organic grade B maple syrup.

Smoked Salmon Frittata

Eggs, salmon, and tomatoes—this recipe is loaded with all the nutrients that you need. The eggs have disease-fighting nutrients like lutein. Your salmon is loaded with omega-3s, a good source of protein, B vitamins, vitamin D, magnesium, and selenium. The tomatoes are also a powerhouse of nutrients from vitamin C, biotin, molybdenum, and vitamin K, copper, potassium, manganese, dietary fiber, vitamin A (in the form of beta-carotene), vitamin B6, folate, niacin, vitamin E, and phosphorus. Sounds like a perfect meal for breakfast or brunch.

3 eggs
2 ounces smoked salmon
1 roma tomato, diced and seeded
1/4 cup chopped onion
1/2 tablespoon chopped parsley leaves
1 tablespoon goat's milk
2 tablespoons olive oil
Salt and pepper to taste

Preheat the oven to 350°F. Break the eggs in a bowl, add goat's milk and seasoning and whisk them. Heat the oil in a cast-iron skillet. Sauté the onions till golden brown; add the diced tomato and add seasoning. Add the salmon and sauté for 2 additional minutes. Pour the egg mixture in the pan and stir gently. Place in the preheated oven and cook for 20–25 minutes.

Homemade Turkey Sausage Patties

Turkey is rich in protein, low in fat, and is a great source of iron, zinc, potassium, phosphorus, vitamin B6, and niacin. It also contains the amino acid tryptophan, selenium, and is lower on the GI index scale.

> 1 pound of ground turkey
> 1 teaspoon of dried sage
> 1/2 teaspoon of fennel seeds
> Dash of cayenne, black pepper, and ground allspice

Mix all ingredients in a bowl. Shape into small 3-inch patties and refrigerate for 2 hours to help form. In a cast-iron skillet on medium heat, cook the patties until completely cooked through on both sides. This would be great with some freshly scrambled eggs.

Honey-Lime Fruit Salad

This easy-to-make breakfast is full of vitamins and antioxidants

> 2 cups chopped seasonal fruits
>   (I use red grapes, kiwis, mandarins, and bananas)
> 1 teaspoon lime juice
> 1 tablespoon organic honey

Combine all the ingredients in a mixing bowl.

Grain-Free Cereals with Apples

> 2 tablespoons chia seeds
> 2 tablespoons of hempseeds
> 2 tablespoons flaxseeds

2 tablespoons pumpkin seeds

1/2 pod vanilla bean, and seeds scooped out, or vanilla extract

1 sliced apple

2 tablespoons of coconut nectar

(Coconut nectar is the perfect healthy liquid sweetener alternative. Organic, Certified Fair Trade, GMO-Free, Gluten-free, vegan. On the Low-glycemic index too)

1/4 teaspoon Himalayan sea salt

2 tablespoons coconut milk

Hot water

Grind the seeds (I grind my seeds in a coffee grinder). Add vanilla beans/extract and sea salt. Pour hot water and coconut butter (if desired) over the seeds. Cover the mixture for about 10 minutes. After mixture thickens add sliced apples

Broccoli and Mushroom Quiche

It's okay to eat cooked cancer-fighting cruciferous vegetables a few times a week.

10 ounces frozen chopped broccoli, cooked and well drained

8 ounces goat cheese crumbles

1/3 cup of onions, chopped

1/3 cup mushrooms, chopped

6 organic, cage free eggs

1 teaspoon of Celtic sea salt

Dash of pepper

Spray a cast iron-skillet. Mix all the ingredients. Bake at 350°F for 35–45 minutes until a knife inserted in the center comes out clean. Let it stand for 10 minutes before cutting.

Side note: Although, I am a strong supporter of almond, coconut milk, and rice milks. Some of my recipes do offer you to use goat cheese instead of cow's milk cheese. Why is that, you might ask.

Nutrition: Goat's milk is a good source of protein, contains less sugar (lactose), 13 percent more calcium, 25 percent more vitamin B6, 47

percent more vitamin A, and 134 percent more potassium than regular cow's milk. Goat cheese also has more vitamin D, vitamin K, thiamine, and niacin, and an equal amount of vitamin A, as cow milk "cheddar." It's also a good source of riboflavin (a B vitamin) and phosphorus too. Even if you have an allergy to milk protein, you may be able to tolerate cheese made from goat's milk because it's formed with shorter amino acid protein chains than cow's milk. Believe it or not, goat's milk has a chemical structure that's similar to that of human breast milk.

Goat's milk is easier to digest than cow's milk. It's naturally homogenized. Goat milk contains less lactose (milk sugar) than cow's milk, which makes it easier on our stomachs simply because we need less of a particular type of enzyme to break down the lactose. If your taste buds can't adjust to almond milk and coconut milk, give goat's milk a try.

Vegetable Quiche

1 bell pepper
2 red onions
1/2 zucchini
3 eggs
1 clove garlic, minced
Fresh parsley leaves (a handful)
3 tablespoon raw, unfiltered coconut oil

Preheat oven to 350°F. Chop vegetables and sauté in 1 1/2 tbsp. oil on medium heat for 3–4 minutes then add to a well-oiled oven-proof dish.

Mix parsley, garlic and eggs in a bowl. Now pour over the vegetables and bake for 25 minutes or until firm in the center.

Breakfast Quinoa with Blueberries

Quinoa is naturally gluten-free and contains iron, B vitamins, magnesium, phosphorus, potassium, calcium, vitamin E, and fiber. Quinoa is a health food superstar. This ancient grain is one of only a few plant foods that are considered a complete protein and has all essential amino acids. Quinoa is a slowly digested carbohydrate, naturally high in dietary fiber, so this makes it a great low-GI option and an awesome choice for diabetics! Can you believe it!?

> 1/2 cup of dry quinoa, rinsed
> 1 cup of unsweetened vanilla almond milk
> 1/2 teaspoon of vanilla extract
> 2 tablespoons of almond butter
> 1/2 teaspoon cinnamon
> 1/2 cup of organic blueberries

Add quinoa, almond milk, and vanilla extract to a saucepan and bring to a boil. Lower heat and simmer with cover on until liquid is absorbed. Fluff quinoa with a fork and let sit uncovered for about a minute. Mix in almond butter, cinnamon, and the blueberries.

Dark Chocolate Chip Blueberry Breakfast Quinoa

> 1/2 cup dry quinoa, rinsed
> 1/2 tablespoons organic coconut oil
> 3/4 cup canned lite coconut milk (reserve more for drizzling)
> 2 teaspoons vanilla extract
> 1/4 teaspoon cinnamon
> A pinch of Celtic sea salt
> 1/4 cup 70 percent dark chocolate chips, shaved
> 1/2 cup fresh blueberries

Melt the coconut oil in a sauce pan. Add the quinoa and coat the oil all over the quinoa and allow it to toast for 2–3 minutes, stirring occasionally. Add the coconut milk, cinnamon, blueberries, and vanilla to your saucepan with quinoa and bring to a boil. Reduce to a simmer, cover, and let cook for 15 minutes until quinoa can be fluffed with a fork.

Put your quinoa into two bowls then sprinkle with your dark chocolate. Dip in!

Apple-Banana Quinoa Breakfast Cups

> 1/2 cup applesauce
> 1 cup mashed banana (about 3 bananas)
> 1 cup cooked quinoa (about 1/2 cup dry)

2 1/2 cups old-fashioned gluten-free oats
1/2 cup almond milk
1/4 cup honey
1 teaspoon vanilla extract
1 teaspoon cinnamon
1 apple, peeled and chopped

Preheat oven to 375°F. Place paper muffin cups in your muffin pan for an easier clean up.

Rinse and cook the quinoa according to the package directions. Once cooked, fluff with a fork. Allow to cook for 5 minutes. Mix all the ingredients in a bowl except the chopped apple.

Fill each of the muffin cups with the quinoa mixture. Top with your chopped apples. Bake for 20–25 minutes. Let cool for 5 minutes and enjoy!

Mini Apple Crisp

1 medium organic apple
1 tablespoon brown sugar
1 tablespoon oats
1/2 teaspoon cinnamon

Heat oven to 350°F. Peel and core the apple and chop into 1/4-inch squares. Mix in a small bowl with sugar, oats, and cinnamon and put into a small baking dish, or line a muffin pan with paper cups. Bake for 15 minutes.

3-Ingredient Pancake Mix

1 banana
2 eggs
1 teaspoon of Ceylon cinnamon
2 tablespoons of Earth Balance butter

Mix all ingredients. Melt butter in a cast-iron skillet. Pour silver-dollar-size amounts of batter in pan. Cook 60 seconds and flip to cook the other side.

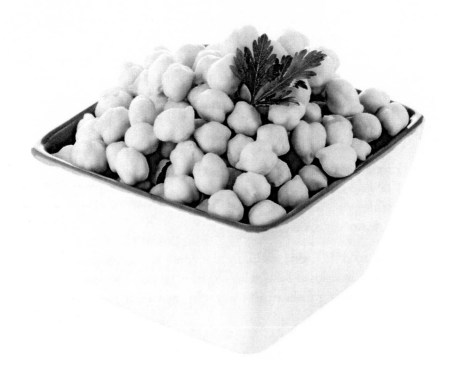

FOR THE LOVE OF CHICKPEA!

Chickpeas are a gluten-free source of protein and fiber. Chickpeas also contain exceptional levels of iron, vitamin B6, and magnesium, vitamin K, folate, phosphorus, zinc, copper, manganese, choline and selenium, and amino acids. Possible health benefits of consuming chickpeas are diabetes (high-fiber diets have lower blood glucose levels), bone health (the iron, phosphate, calcium, magnesium, manganese, zinc, and vitamin K content present in chickpeas all contribute to building and maintaining bone structure and strength), blood pressure (low-sodium intake is essential to lowering blood pressure), heart health (high fiber, potassium, vitamin C and vitamin B6 content, coupled with the lack of cholesterol found in chickpeas, all support heart health), cancer (selenium is a mineral that plays a role in liver enzyme function and helps detoxify some cancer-causing compounds in the body; additionally, selenium prevents inflammation and also decreases tumor growth rates), lowers cholesterol, fights inflammation, and aids in your digestion and regularity! So why not eat this *superfood* up?

Amino acids are the building blocks of proteins and are extremely important in ensuring that the body functions properly. Some, known as nonessential amino acids, can be produced by the body when they are needed. Essential amino acids, however, cannot be made in the body and therefore must be consumed in the diet.

Simply Roasted Chickpea

> 2 tablespoons extra-virgin olive oil
> 1 tablespoon ground cumin
> 1 teaspoon garlic powder
> 1/2 teaspoon of chili powder
> Pinch of Celtic sea salt
> Pinch of ground black pepper
> Pinch of crushed red pepper
> 1 can (15 oz.) chickpeas, drained and rinsed

Preheat oven to 350°F degrees. Place the chickpeas in a large bowl and toss with the remaining ingredients until evenly coated. Spread the chickpeas in an even layer on a baking sheet and bake until crisp, about 30 to 45 minutes. Note: every 10 minutes, shake your pan to move the chickpeas around.

Roasted Pumpkin Spice Chickpeas

> 1 can chickpeas rinsed and drained
> 1/3 cup can pumpkin puree
> 3 T honey
> 1 teaspoon Ceylon cinnamon
> 1/4 teaspoon ground cloves
> 1/4 teaspoon ground ginger
> 1/4 teaspoon ground nutmeg

Preheat oven to 350°F degrees. Place the chickpeas in a large bowl and toss with the remaining ingredients until evenly coated. Spread the chickpeas in an even layer on a baking sheet and bake until crisp, about 30 to 45 minutes. Note: every 10 minutes, shake your pan to move the chickpeas around.

Three-Spice Oven-Roasted Chickpeas

2 cans (15 oz) chickpeas, also known as garbanzo beans, thoroughly drained and rinsed (about 3 cups)
2 tablespoons coconut oil
1 teaspoon ground cumin
1 teaspoon chili powder
1/2 teaspoon cayenne pepper
1/2 teaspoon sea salt

Heat the oven to 400°F and arrange a rack in the middle. Place the chickpeas in a large bowl and toss with the remaining ingredients until evenly coated. Spread the chickpeas in an even layer on a baking sheet and bake until crisp, about 30 to 45 minutes. Note: every 10 minutes, shake your pan to move the chickpeas around.

Chili-Lime Roasted Chickpeas

2 15-ounce cans chickpeas (also called garbanzo beans), drained, rinsed and blotted dry
1 tablespoon chili powder
2 tablespoon olive oil
The juice from half of a freshly squeezed lime
Pinch of Himalayan sea salt
2 teaspoon cumin
1 teaspoons finely grated lime zest

Preheat oven to 400°F. Place the chickpeas in a large bowl and toss with all the ingredients, except for the lime zest, until evenly coated. Spread the chickpeas in an even layer on a nonaluminum baking pan or in a large cast-iron skillet. Bake until crisp, about 40 to 45 minutes. Sprinkle the lime zest on the chickpeas after cooked. Note: every 10 minutes, shake your pan to move the chickpeas around.

BBQ-Roasted Chickpeas

1 15-ounce can chick peas, drained and rinsed
1 teaspoon chipotle chili power
1 teaspoon garlic powder
1 teaspoon smoked paprika

1/2 teaspoon Himalayan sea salt

1 teaspoon coconut of melted oil or EVOO

Place the chickpeas in a large bowl and toss with the remaining ingredients until evenly coated. Spread the chickpeas in an even layer on a rimmed baking sheet and bake until crisp, about 30 to 45 minutes. Note: every 10 minutes, shake your pan to move the chickpeas around.

Roasted Cinnamon-Honey Chickpeas

1 can 15-ounce garbanzo beans, rinsed and drained

1/2 teaspoon ground cinnamon

1 tablespoon coconut oil

1 tablespoon honey

Preheat oven to 400°F. Place the chickpeas in a large bowl and toss with all the ingredients, except the honey, until evenly coated. Spread the chickpeas in an even layer on a baking sheet and bake until crisp, about 30 to 45 minutes. Note: every 10 minutes, shake your pan to move the chickpeas around.

Fire-Roasted Tomato-Quinoa Penne Pasta with Crispy Chickpeas and Zucchini

1 can fire-roasted, diced tomatoes, not drained

1 cup uncooked organic zucchini, diced

1 can (15 oz) cooked chickpeas

2 tablespoon goat's cheese, crumbled

2 cloves garlic, minced

2 tablespoon olive oil

8 oz quinoa penne pasta

Celtic sea salt and pepper to taste

Cook the quinoa pasta according to package; drain and set aside. Meanwhile in a large cast-iron skillet, heat 1 tablespoon of olive oil and sauté zucchini, garlic, and chickpeas over medium-high heat for about 12 minutes. After the chickpeas have cooked and become browned and crispy, add the cooked pasta with zucchini, roasted tomatoes, and chickpeas. Mix well. Cook additional 5 minutes to allow and blend all the flavorings together. Season to taste and sprinkle goat cheese crumbles.

Curried Chickpea Stew with Brown Rice Pilaf

Pilaf:

1 tablespoon canola oil
1 cup finely chopped onion
1 cup uncooked brown rice
1/2 teaspoon ground turmeric
1 (3-inch) cinnamon stick
1 garlic clove, minced
1 tabs of tomato paste
1 2/3 cups water
1 bay leaf

Stew:

1 tablespoon EVOO
2 cups chopped onion
1 tablespoon grated, peeled fresh ginger
1 teaspoon ground cumin
1 teaspoon ground coriander
3/4 teaspoon ground turmeric
1/4 teaspoon ground red pepper
4 garlic cloves, minced
1 (3-inch) cinnamon stick
2 1/2 cups water
1 cup diced carrot
1/4 teaspoon kosher salt
1 (15 oz) can chickpeas (garbanzo beans), rinsed and drained
1 (14.5 oz) can fire-roasted, crushed tomatoes, undrained (such as Muir Glen)
1/2 cup plain nonfat goat's milk yogurt
1/4 cup chopped fresh cilantro

To prepare pilaf, heat a large iron skillet over medium heat. Melt 1 tablespoon of oil to coat the pan. Add 1 cup chopped onion; cook for 6 minutes, stirring frequently. Add rice and the next 4 ingredients (through garlic); cook for 1 minute, stirring constantly. Add 1 2/3 cups water, tomato paste, and bay leaf; bring to a boil. Cover, reduce heat, and simmer for 45 minutes. Let stand for 5 minutes. Discard cinnamon and bay leaf. Cover with a lid to keep warm.

To prepare the stew, heat a large dutch oven over medium-high heat. Add 1 tablespoon oil and coat pan. Add 2 cups onion; sauté for 6 minutes. Add ginger and the next 7 ingredients; cook for 1 minute, stirring constantly. Add 2 1/2 cups water, carrot, 1/4 teaspoon salt, chickpeas, and tomatoes; bring to a boil. Cover, reduce heat, and simmer for 20 minutes or until carrots are tender and sauce is slightly thick. Discard cinnamon stick.

Place 1 cup rice mixture into each of 4 bowls; spoon 1 1/4 cups chickpea mixture over rice. Top each serving with 2 tablespoons yogurt and 1 tablespoon cilantro.

Chickpea and Butternut Squash Stew

1 large onion, chopped
2 tablespoons olive oil
Black pepper and Celtic sea salt
2 medium zucchini (about 1 pound total),
    cut into 1 1/2-inch bite-size pieces
1 butternut squash (about 1 1/2 pounds),
    cut into 1/2-inch bite-size pieces
1 15.5-ounce can diced tomatoes
1 15.5-ounce can chickpeas, rinsed and drained
1 teaspoon ground ginger
1 teaspoon ground coriander
1 cup cooked quinoa or cooked brown rice
Fresh cilantro leaves, for serving

Heat the oil in a cast-iron skillet over medium heat. Add the onion and 1/4 teaspoon salt and cook, stirring constantly until tender, 6 to 8 minutes. Add the zucchini and cook, stirring occasionally until crisp-tender, 3 to 5 minutes. Add the squash, tomatoes, chickpeas, ginger, coriander, and 1/4 teaspoon each of salt and pepper. Cook covered, stirring occasionally until the squash is tender, 15 to 18 minutes.

Meanwhile, cook the quinoa or brown rice according to package directions.

Place 1 cup of your cooked brown rice or quinoa into bowls; spoon 1 1/4 cups chickpea and butternut squash stew mixture over rice. Top with a sprinkle of cilantro leaves.

Chickpea Curry

> 1 tablespoon olive oil
> 1 15-ounce can chickpeas, drained and rinsed
> 1 large onion chopped
> 1 1/2 teaspoons ginger powder
> 1 teaspoon cumin
> 1/2 teaspoon salt
> 1/8 teaspoon black pepper
> 5 cloves garlic, minced
> 5 teaspoons curry powder
> 1 large tomato chopped
> Good pinch of cinnamon
> Pinch of oregano
> 2/3 cup water

Heat oil in a cast-iron skillet; add onion and cook until tender. Add garlic; cook additional for 1 minute. Add ginger and curry, stir to mix and cook an additional 2 minutes. Add chickpeas, salt, pepper, cumin, cinnamon, water, stir to mix. Cook an additional 5 minutes. Next add your tomato and oregano, stir to mix. Cover your pan and simmer until tomatoes are cooked down, stirring often to prevent sticking.

Depending how thick you like it, remove lid and continue cooking to remove some of the excess liquid or until desired thickness is reached.

Chickpea Soup

> 3 15-ounce cans chickpeas, rinsed
> 3 tablespoons olive oil
> 2 large onions, diced
> 4 garlic cloves, minced

1 sprig thyme
1/2 cup dry white wine
4 cups vegetable broth
Himalayan sea salt
Flat-leaf parsley and fresh tarragon leaves (for garnish)

Heat oil in a cast-iron skillet over medium heat. Add onions, garlic, and thyme sprig; cook, stirring occasionally until onions are soft, 10-15 minutes. Add chickpeas and wine. Bring to a steady simmer; cook until wine is reduced by half, about 2 additional minutes. Add broth and reduce heat; cover and simmer until chickpeas are very soft, about 30 minutes for canned. Discard thyme sprig.

Working in batches, purée chickpea mixture in a blender or with a handheld immersion blender. Blend until smooth. Season with salt.

Chickpea Stew

4 tablespoons coconut oil, divided
2 skinless, boneless chicken thighs (preferably organic, antibiotic- and hormone-free)
Himalayan sea salt
3 large garlic cloves, minced
2 tablespoons ground cumin
2 tablespoons tomato paste
3/4 teaspoon crushed red pepper flakes
2 bay leaves
2 15-ounce cans chickpeas, rinsed and drained
1/2 cup chopped roasted red peppers drained from a jar
2 tablespoons (or more) fresh lemon juice

Heat 2 tablespoon oil in a dutch oven over medium-high heat. Season chicken with salt; add to your dutch oven and cook, turning once until browned, 8–10 minutes. Transfer chicken to a plate. Add garlic and cook, stirring often until soft, 2 minutes. Add cumin, tomato paste, and red pepper flakes; stir until a smooth paste forms, about 1 minute. Add the chicken back with the bay leaves and 4 cups of water. Scrape up any browned bits. Bring to a boil; reduce heat to medium low and simmer, uncovered, occasionally stirring until chicken is tender, about 20 minutes.

Transfer chicken to a clean plate. Add chickpeas to pot; bring to a simmer and cook for 5 minutes. Shred chicken; add to stew. Add red peppers. Stir in remaining 2 tablespoon oil and 2 tablespoon lemon juice; simmer for 1 minute. Season with salt and more lemon juice if desired.

You can eat this over brown rice or quinoa to make it a complete, fulfilling meal.

Fried Chickpeas

2 teaspoons smoked paprika
1 teaspoon cayenne pepper
6 tablespoons extra-virgin olive oil
2 15-ounce cans chickpeas, rinsed, drained, patted very dry
Kosher salt
2 teaspoons finely grated lime zest

Combine paprika and cayenne in a small bowl and set aside. Heat oil in a cast-iron skillet over medium-high heat. Working in 2 batches, add chickpeas to skillet and sauté, stirring frequently until golden and crispy, 15–20 minutes. Using a slotted spoon, transfer chickpeas to paper towels to get excess oil off. Transfer to a bowl. Sprinkle paprika mixture over; toss to coat. Season to taste with salt. Toss with lime zest and serve. You can eat this over a bowl of brown rice or quinoa.

Spicy Crunchy Chickpeas

2 tablespoons olive oil
1 teaspoon cinnamon
1 teaspoon cumin
1 teaspoon allspice
1 teaspoon Celtic sea salt
1/2 teaspoon pepper
2 15 1/2-ounces cans chickpeas, rinsed, drained, patted dry

Preheat oven to 400°F. Line a large rimmed baking sheet with parchment paper. In a large bowl, combine olive oil, cinnamon, cumin, allspice, salt, and pepper. Add chickpeas and toss to coat. Pour the chickpeas mixture onto your baking sheet and roast, stirring or shaking baking sheet every 10 minutes until chickpeas are browned and crunchy, 45 to 50 minutes. Transfer to a bowl and let cool before serving.

Easy Hummus with Tahini

> 1 15-ounce can of chickpeas, drained (reserve
> 1 tablespoon of the liquid)
> 1 small garlic clove, smashed
> 1 tablespoon fresh lemon juice
> 1/4 cup tahini
> Extra-virgin olive oil
> Pinch of sweet, smoked paprika
> Kosher salt

In a food processor, combine the chickpeas with the liquid, garlic, lemon juice, and tahini and puree to a chunky paste. Scrape down the side of the bowl. Add 2 tablespoons of olive oil and the paprika and puree until smooth. Season the hummus with salt; drizzle with olive oil.

Chickpea, Avocado, and Crumbled Goat Cheese Salad

> 1 can chickpeas, rinsed and drained
> 2 avocados, pitted and chopped
> 1/3 cup chopped cilantro
> 2 tablespoons green onion
> 1/3 cup crumbled goat cheese
> Juice of 1 lime
> Salt and black pepper to taste

In a medium bowl, combine chickpeas, avocado, cilantro, green onion, feta cheese, and lime juice. Stir until mixed well. Season with salt and pepper.

Quinoa Chickpea and Avocado Salad

 1 cup quartered grape tomatoes
 15-ounce can garbanzo beans, rinsed and drained
 1 cup cooked quinoa
 2 tablespoon red onion, minced
 2 tablespoon cilantro, minced
 1 1/2 limes, juiced
 Kosher salt and fresh pepper to taste
 1 cup diced cucumber
 4 oz diced avocado (1 medium Hass)

Combine all the ingredients except for avocado and cucumber; season with salt and pepper to taste. Keep refrigerated until ready to serve. Just before serving, add cucumber and avocado.

Tuna and Chickpea Salad

 2 15-ounce cans chickpeas, drained and rinsed
 1 12-ounce can chunk light tuna packed in water, drained
 2 cups cherry tomatoes, halved (quartered if large)
 1/2 cup of red bell pepper, diced
 1 shallot, finely chopped
 1/4 cup finely chopped fresh parsley
 3 tablespoons olive oil
 3 tablespoons lemon juice
 Celtic sea salt and pepper

Lay down a bed of romaine lettuce. In a large bowl, combine beans, tuna, tomatoes, red bell pepper, shallot, and parsley. Drizzle oil and lemon juice over mixture. Toss well; season with salt and pepper. You can eat this over a nice bed of romaine salad.

Greek Salad with Chickpeas and Sardines

 3 tablespoons lemon juice
 2 tablespoons extra-virgin olive oil
 1 clove garlic, minced

2 teaspoons dried oregano
1/2 teaspoon freshly ground pepper
3 medium tomatoes, cut into large chunks
1 large English cucumber, cut into large chunks
1 15-ounce can chickpeas, rinsed
1/3 cup crumbled goat cheese
1/4 cup thinly sliced red onion
2 tablespoons sliced Kalamata olives
2 4-ounce cans sardines with bones packed in olive oil or water, drained

Whisk lemon juice, oil, garlic, oregano, and pepper in a large bowl until well combined. Add tomatoes, cucumber, chickpeas, feta, onion and olives; gently toss to combine. Divide the salad among 4 plates and top with sardines.

Cold Zucchini Noodles with Chickpeas and Tomatoes Salad

2 large zucchini, peeled and made into noodles
1 can chickpeas, rinsed well
1 pint tomatoes, halved
3 tablespoon extra-virgin olive oil
2 cloves garlic, finely minced
1 lemon, juiced
Salt and pepper to taste

Make your zucchini noodles. Add the halved tomatoes and rinsed chickpeas with the zucchini noodles. Toss with the olive oil, minced garlic, lemon juice, and salt and pepper to taste. Let marinate in the fridge for at least 30 minutes and ideally several hours before serving.

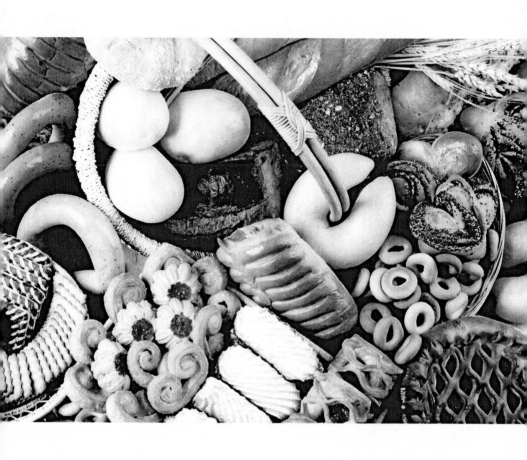

BREADS, COOKIES, AND CAKES: OH MY!

I collected many amazing gluten-free, grain-free bread recipes designed from my creative expression and adapted from other recipe gurus expressed in my own words. These will delight your taste buds and put a smile upon your face.

Coconut flour is one of the healthiest gluten-free, grain-free flours, and it's low in carbs too. It contains fat from coconut oil, which is awesome for your thyroid and is mostly medium-chain saturated fatty acids (MCTS). MCTS have been shown to improve your metabolism and are used for energy and is very low in omega-6. Omega-6 can be an inflammatory to your body when consumed in high amounts. Although gluten- and grain-free, nut and seed flours tend to have more omega-6; that's why you will see more coconut flour recipe in my book. Nut and seed flours are still a better alternative than store-bought bread that is loaded with dough conditioners, GMOs, corn oil, soybean oil, preservatives, high-fructose corn syrup, artificial flavors and coloring, added sugars. You can store coconut flour in an airtight container at room temperature. The shelf life is few couple of months, or you can freeze and bring to room temperature before using in a recipe.

Blueberry Coconut Cups

 1 cup coconut butter
 1 cup blueberries
 1 cup virgin coconut oil
 1/3 cup raw honey
 1/4 cup shredded unsweetened coconut
 1/4 cup coconut flour

Heat your blueberries and honey in a small saucepan over medium heat. Mix and allow the blueberries to break down and pop. Once your blueberries have popped, add your coconut oil and coconut butter. Stir all together. Remove from heat and add your shredded coconut and coconut flour. Line your muffin tin with paper muffin liners, pour mixture into each cup to a height that you prefer then place in freezer for 20 minutes.

Microwave "Bread"

 2 tablespoon nondairy or nonsoy salted butter,
     melted and slightly cooled
 1 large egg
 1 tablespoon coconut flour
 1/4 teaspoon aluminum free baking powder

In a medium bowl, mix the ingredients until blended well. You want a smooth consistency. Pour your mixture into a medium size micro-wavable glass bowl. Microwave on high for 90 seconds. Bread will puff up while "cooking" then deflate. It will look like a muffin. Make sure it appears set; otherwise, microwave 30 more seconds—90 seconds is generally enough time. You can overcook it and make it very dry.

 With a small knife, gently loosen the bread edges and remove from the bowl onto a plate. Slice into and top with your favorite toppings.

Coconut Flour Tortillas

 2 cups of coconut flour
 1 teaspoon aluminum-free baking powder

2 egg whites
2 tablespoons of coconut milk or water
1 tablespoon EVOO

Mix all the ingredients, except the EVOO, until smooth. Grease your cast iron skillet with EVOO.

Pour 2 tablespoons of your batter into center of pan, tilt the pan around to spread the batter into a large circle, almost covering the entire pan. Cook for 30 seconds. Be careful; wait until edges are brown to flip. Once you flip, cook another 30 seconds. *Baam!* You've just made yourself a coconut flour tortilla.

Almond Flour tortillas

2 cups of almond flour
2 eggs
1 teaspoon olive oil
1/2 teaspoon sea salt

Mix well; this should make 5 tortillas. Divide into 5 balls and spread on parchment paper. Oven to 350°F, 8 minutes. You can also make this in a cast-iron skillet, if you want them crispy. Just oil your pan, take each ball individually, shape into a tortilla, place in your heated medium-heated cast-iron skillet, and cook for 30–45 seconds on each side.

Almond Bread

This is a nice bread to eat in the morning with fresh blueberries. Its low-carb, gluten- and grain-free.

2.5 cups almond meal
1.5 teaspoon arrowroot powder
1 tablespoon Aluminum-free baking powder
1 tablespoon raw honey
3 eggs
1 teaspoon sea salt
1/2 teaspoon apple cider vinegar

Preheat your oven to 300°F. In a bowl, mix all your dry ingredients. In a second bowl, mix all your wet ingredients. Combine the two mixtures, grease the loaf pan, and then line the loaf pan with a long piece of parchment paper where it slightly over laps the edges of the pan. Grease the parchment paper too. Pour into a greased loaf pan. Bake for 45–55 minutes. You can check the doneness by sticking a toothpick in the center. By placing the parchment paper in your loaf pan, this will make the bread pop out easily.

Corn Bread

1 cup coconut flour
1/4 cup raw honey
1 teaspoon Celtic sea salt
3 1/2 teaspoon baking powder
5 eggs
1/2 cup vanilla almond milk
1/3 cup coconut oil
1 can (15 oz) baby corn, well drained and chopped fine

Preheat oven to 400°F. Lightly grease a cast-iron skillet. Place your cast-iron skillet in the oven to heat up while you're making the mixture. Drain baby corn and chop into small pieces. In a large bowl, combine all your ingredients and mix well. Pour batter into your heated cast-iron skillet. Bake in your preheated oven for 20 to 25 minutes or until a toothpick inserted into the center of the cornbread comes out clean.

Coconut Flour Flatbread

1 large egg
1 tablespoon coconut flour
1 tablespoon goat cheese
1/8 teaspoon baking soda
1/8 teaspoon baking powder
2 pinches of Himalayan sea salt
2 tablespoon of coconut milk
2 tablespoons of nondairy butter

Mix all the ingredients in a large bowl. Melt a tablespoon of butter in the cast-iron skillet over medium-low heat. Pour two small sandwich-sized "pancakes" into your cast-iron skillet. It will spread just a tad bit. Once you see the tops start to bubble and brown on the bottom, flip; cook an additional 30–45 seconds. You can add Italian spices and make this your crust for a pizza!

Almond Buns

> 3/4 cup almond flour
> 2 large eggs
> 5 tablespoon unsalted nondairy butter
> 1.5 teaspoon baking powder

Combine the dry ingredients in a bowl; mix in your eggs. Add your melted butter to the mixture and stir well. This should make 6 muffins. Lay on a parchment paper and spray the paper with olive oil spray. Bake for 12–17 minutes at 350°F. Every oven is different, so keep an eye out on your buns. Once done, transfer to a wire rack to cool.

Cinnamon Sweet Coconut Bread

> 2 large eggs
> 1 1/4 cups coconut milk
> 1 teaspoon vanilla extract
> 2 1/2 cups coconut flour
> 1/4 teaspoon Celtic sea salt or pink Himalayan sea salt
> 2 teaspoons aluminum-free baking powder
> 1 to 2 teaspoons ground cinnamon
> 1 cup granulated sugar
> 1.5 cups sweetened flaked coconut
> 6 tablespoons unsalted butter, melted
> EVOO nonstick cooking spray for baking pan

Heat oven to 350°F. In a small bowl, whisk together eggs, milk and vanilla. In a medium bowl, sift together coconut flour, salt, baking powder, and cinnamon. Add sugar and coconut and stir to mix. Make a hole in the center and pour in egg mixture then stir wet and dry ingredients together until just combined. Add butter and stir until just smooth try not to not to over mix.

Butter and sprinkle with flour a 9×5-inch loaf pan and coat it with a nonstick spray. You can also line your loaf pan with parchment paper to make it an easy pull-out. Spread batter in pan and bake until a toothpick inserted into the center comes out clean, anywhere from 1 to 1 1/4 hours. Cool in pan five minutes before turning onto a cooling rack.

Serve in thick slices, toasted, with butter and confectioners' sugar.

Coffee Cake

   1 cup coconut flour
   1/2 teaspoon Celtic sea salt
   1 teaspoon ground cinnamon
   8 large eggs
   1 teaspoon baking soda
   1/2 cup plain coconut milk yogurt
   5 tablespoons unsalted butter or coconut oil, melted
   1/2 cup raw honey
   1 tablespoon vanilla extract

Topping:

   1 1/2 cups nuts (almonds, pecans, cashews, etc.)
   2 teaspoons cinnamon
   4 tablespoons raw honey
   4 tablespoons unsalted butter or coconut oil,
       cold, cut into tablespoons

Preheat oven to 325°F and adjust rack to middle position. Place all the batter ingredients in a food processor and blend until smooth. Pour batter into a buttered 8×8-inch baking dish. Next, place nuts, cinnamon, honey, and butter in the food processor and pulse until the nuts looks coarsely chopped and the ingredients are combined. Drop spoonfuls of topping over batter, and then using a butter knife, swirl the topping into the top layer of the batter. Bake for 40–45 minutes until golden brown. Let cool for 20 minutes. Cut and serve.

Cranberry Orange Coconut Flour Bread

 6 eggs
 1/2 cup coconut flour
 1/4 cup raw honey
 1/4 cup freshly squeezed orange juice
 1/4 cup cranberries
 1 teaspoon vanilla
 1/2 teaspoon cinnamon
 1 teaspoon baking soda
 Orange zest (however much you're able to get is fine)

Preheat oven to 350°F. Mix all the ingredients except cranberries together in a large bowl with a hand mixer. Next, add the cranberries. Pour the mix into a loaf pan lined with parchment paper. Bake for 35–40 minutes until a toothpick inserted into the center comes out clean.

Coconut Flour French Toast

 8 slices coconut flour bread, about 1/2 inch thick
 2 large eggs
 1 tablespoon almond milk
 1/2 teaspoon ground cinnamon
 2 teaspoon butter or coconut oil

Preheat oven to 200°F. You want your bread to be a bit dry and workable. Arrange slices of bread on a wire rack set over a baking sheet and place in oven. Let dry out for about 1 hour.

In a medium bowl, whisk together eggs, cream, and cinnamon until well combined. Pour your batter into a large shallow dish. Allow your bread slices to sit for about 30 seconds on each side to soak up the liquid mixture. Meanwhile, heat a cast-iron skillet over medium heat. Add butter and cook until butter just begins to brown, swirling to coat the bottom of the pan. As you're removing your bread from the batter, shake lightly to remove excess batter. Place in skillet and cook until golden brown on both sides, 2 to 3 minutes per side. Repeat until done.

Crisp Rosemary-Parmesan Flatbread Recipe

2 cups almond flour
2 tablespoons unsalted butter, chilled and cubed
1/4 cup goat cheese, grated (plus more for serving)
1 egg white
1/2 teaspoon McCormick dried rosemary

Preheat oven to 350°F. Add all the ingredients to a food processor; pulse until well combined. Place dough on parchment, pressing down firmly with your hand to make it flat. Place another piece of parchment on top and roll out thinly with a rolling pin.

Remove top piece of parchment and prick dough all over with a fork. Place parchment with dough on baking sheet and bake until golden, about 15 minutes or until light-golden brown.

Let cool on a wire rack.

Pumpkin Bread

1 cup blanched almond flour
1/4 teaspoon celtic sea salt
1/2 teaspoon baking soda
1 tablespoon ground cinnamon
1 teaspoon nutmeg
1/2 teaspoon cloves
1/2 cup roasted pumpkin
2 tablespoons honey
3 large eggs

In a food processor, combine the dry ingredients; pulse until well combined. Next, add your wet ingredients and pulse until combined. Pour your batter into a mini loaf pan. Bake at 350°F for 35–45 minutes. Allow to cool for 1 hour.

Banana Nut Bread

2 bananas, mashed
1 1/2 cups brown rice flour

1 teaspoon baking powder
3/4 cup brown rice, old-fashioned
3 egg whites
1/2 cup raisins
1/3 cup applesauce
1/3 cup chopped up Brazil nuts
1 teaspoon cinnamon

Combine all wet ingredients: banana, applesauce, eggs, and vanilla. Next, combine the remaining dry ingredients in a separate bowl. Add the dry mixture to wet mixture slowly and stir until the two are just combined.

Spray loaf pan with nonstick spray and pour in the cake mixture. Bake at 350°F until the top is brown, 30–45 minutes. Stick a toothpick in the center to check for doneness. Allow to cool for 1 hour.

Gluten-Free Oatmeal Chip Bars

1/2 cup packed brown sugar
4 eggs
3 medium mashed ripe bananas
1 cup almond butter
6 cups of gluten-free old-fashioned oats
1 cup butterscotch chips
1 cup of semisweet chocolate chips

In a large bowl, beat brown sugar and eggs until well blended. Add bananas, almond butter, and blend. Stir in oats and the butterscotch and chocolate chips.

Spread the batter on a baking pan coasted with cooking spray. Bake at 350°F for 20 minutes until edges begin to brown. Cool completely on a wire rack. Cut into bars; it makes about 3 dozen bars.

Apricot Squares

2 cups gluten-free old-fashioned oats
1/4 cup ground flaxseed
3/4 teaspoon ground cinnamon

1/4 teaspoon ground cloves

1/4 teaspoon salt

1/2 cup almond butter

1/4 cup raw honey

1 teaspoon vanilla extract

1/2 cup finely chopped apricots

Preheat your oven to 350°F. Coat your 8×8-inch pan with spray. First mix the dry ingredients in a bowl. Next, mix the wet ingredients in a separate bowl. Add to the dry ingredients your wet ingredients and mix to combine. Mix in the apricots until well combined. Press the mixture firmly into your prepared pan. Bake for 25 minutes or until the edges are browned. Let it cool completely before cutting into eight bars. Store in an airtight container.

Sesame Squares

1/3 cup honey

1/3 cup almond butter

3/4 cup nonfat dry goat's milk

2 tablespoons of ground flaxseed meal

3/4 cup sesame seeds

1/4 cup raisins

1/4 cup shredded coconut

Mix all your ingredients in a bowl and combine well. Spread your mixture into an 8×8-inch baking pan and refrigerate for four hours. Cut into 1-inch squares.

Almond Butter Freezer Fudge

2 cups raw creamy almond butter (unsalted)

1/2 cup coconut oil, room temp

3 tablespoons raw honey

1 teaspoon fine Himalayan sea salt

Mix all the ingredients together in a medium bowl until well combined. Pour your mixture into a square baking dish lined with parchment then smooth out with a spatula and freeze until solid (about an hour). Remove the fudge by lifting the paper out of the pan; then cut into squares.

Buttercup Bars

    3/4 cup almond butter
    4 tablespoons coconut oil (divided)
    4 tablespoons raw honey (divided)
    1/2 cup unsweetened cocoa powder
    2 tablespoons chocolate chips

Slowly and carefully heat almond butter and 2 tablespoons coconut oil over medium-low heat. Once melted, remove from heat and add 2 tablespoons honey. Stir until well combined. Pour into a small baking dish (8×8 or similar) and smooth out in one single smooth layer. Place in the freezer for at least 15 minutes.

Heat 2 tablespoons coconut oil over low heat and add cocoa powder. Remove from heat and add remaining 2 tablespoons honey. Spread chocolate mixture over frozen almond butter mixture. Sprinkle with chocolate chips. Place in the freezer for at least 30 minutes.

Remove the dish from the freezer and let warm slightly. Cut into squares and serve immediately or return them to the freezer.

Chocolate Coconut Almond Candy

    2/3 cup unsweetened cocoa powder
    2/3 cup sugar
    3/4 unsweetened dried shredded coconut or flakes
    1/2 cup sliced almonds
    1 cup coconut oil (melted)
    1 1/2 teaspoons vanilla extract
    1/2 teaspoon almond extract

Mix all ingredients well in a bowl. Add extra coconut or almonds if desired.

Pour candy into a glass pan or cookie sheet and refrigerate until firm. Break into pieces and keep refrigerated.

Almond Butter Cookies

1/2 cup pitted, dried Medjool dates, stems removed
1 1/2 cups whole raw almonds
1/4 cup almond butter
2 tablespoons maple syrup
1/4 teaspoon almond extract
1/4 teaspoon cinnamon
1 cup dried cherries
1/2 cup rolled oats

Line your baking sheet with parchment. Blend first 6 ingredients in a food processor until smooth. You may need to add 1 teaspoon of water in batches to help the mixture hold together. Next, add in cherries and oats. Pulse a few times.

Scooping a tablespoonful, roll dough into balls; place on baking sheet that can fit in your fridge. Flatten slightly. Cover with plastic wrap; refrigerate until firm, about 1 hour. Store between sheets of parchment paper in an airtight container in the refrigerator for up to 1 week.

Caramelized Coconut Chips

1 cup unsweetened coconut chips
1/4 teaspoon sea salt
Pinch of cinnamon

Mix the sea salt and cinnamon in a small bowl. Heat a nonstick pan over medium-high heat for about 2 minutes. Add the coconut flakes and distribute evenly so they form a shallow layer in the bottom of the pan. Stir frequently—they begin to crisp and turn brown pretty quickly. Once the flakes have reached a nice looking level of "toastiness," remove from the heat. Once it cools, add your coconut flakes to your sea salt and cinnamon mixture. You can store this in an airtight container in the fridge.

Coffee-Coconut Ice Cream

This excellent-tasting creamy coffee ice cream is made with coconut milk, pure vanilla extract, and raw sugar. Yum!

    2 13.5-ounce cans of quality full-fat coconut milk
        (roughly 3 1/2 cups)
    3/4 cup raw sugar, depending on preferred sweetness
        (I used 1/2 cup)
    3/4 cup strong brewed coffee or decaf if you prefer
    1.5 teaspoon pure vanilla extract

Combine coconut milk, coffee, and raw sugar in a small saucepan over medium heat and mix until combined, roughly about 5 minutes.

Remove from heat and mix in the vanilla. Transfer to a bowl to let cool completely in the fridge—at least 6 hours or overnight. Transfer to ice cream maker and prepare according to manufacturer instructions. This delicious recipe should keep for 1 week in the freezer.

Date, Prune, and Fig Coconut Rolls

    1/2 cup dried dates
    3/4 cup dried figs
    4 dried prunes
    1/2 cup walnuts
    1 tbsp. coconut oil
    1/2 cup fresh shredded coconut

Pulse everything together in a food processor, except the shredded coconuts. Blend until mixture looks like a paste. Using a teaspoon, scoop a small about of the mixture, roll between the palms of your hands to form a little ball. Roll in coconut shavings. Store in an airtight container and place them in the refrigerator.

Homemade Microwavable Popcorn

    A brown paper bag
    1/4 cup of popping corn

1 teaspoon extra-virgin olive oil
Popcorn salt to taste

Pour the raw, hard popcorn in the brown paper bag. Add your salt; shake salt all over popcorn and add a teaspoon of olive oil. Fold the top of the bag over twice and set microwave to 3 to 5 minutes, depending on your microwave power. I have a popcorn button on my microwave, so it takes all the "timed" guesswork out for me. Add extra seasonings if you wish.

Dark Chocolate Coconut Figs

5 dried figs
1/2 ounce dark chocolate

Sprinkle some coarse Celtic sea salt and shredded coconut. Lay a piece of parchment paper on a plate. Heat dark chocolate in a small bowl in the microwave at 20 second intervals. Stir often and heat until *just* melted (chocolate burns easily in the microwave). Dip 1/2 fig in chocolate, put on plate, and dust with salt. Refrigerate for 1/2 hour and serve.

Dark Chocolate Coconut Apricot Bites

5 dried apricots
1/2 ounce dark chocolate

Sprinkle some coarse Celtic sea salt and shredded coconut. Lay a piece of parchment paper on a plate. Heat dark chocolate in a small bowl in the microwave at 20 second intervals. Stir often and heat until *just* melted (chocolate burns easily in the microwave). Dip 1/2 apricot in the chocolate, put on plate, and dust with salt. Refrigerate for 1/2 hour and serve.

Sesame Squares

1/3 cup raw honey
1/3 cup Almond butter
3/4 cup sesame seeds

1/4 cup raisins
1/4 cup shredded coconut

Mix all the ingredients in a large. Spread the mixture into an 8×8-inch baking pan and refrigerate for 4 hours. Cut into 1-inch squares.

No-Bake Oatmeal Bites

1 cup dry quick oats
2/3 cup coconut flakes
1/2 cup almond butter
1/2 cup dark chocolate chips
1/3 cup raw honey
1 teaspoon vanilla

Mix all ingredients; form into 1 inch balls. Place balls in refrigerator and snack away.

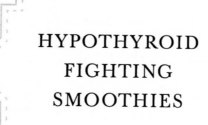

HYPOTHYROID FIGHTING SMOOTHIES

All my smoothie recipes are vegan, gluten-free, and dairy-free. I've added fifteen different drink and smoothie recipes to help you shed a few pounds, jump-start your metabolism, and get that thyroid in motion. Let's get to sipping! You can also replace a smoothie with a meal.

Autumn Pumpkin Smoothie Supreme

This smoothie packs a nutritional punch. It provides antioxidants and fiber from the pumpkin, protein from the almond butter, and potassium from the banana. Add a tablespoon of flaxseed oil or hempseed oil for your omega-3s! This *super-easy-to-make* pumpkin spice smoothie is an awesome way to slurp up the great flavors of autumn.

    1/2 cup pumpkin puree
    1/2 cup canned coconut cream (or sub almond/coconut milk)
    2 tablespoons almond butter
    1 banana
    2 dates, soaked overnight to soften
    1 teaspoon cinnamon

Place all the ingredients into a blender and puree until smooth. Serve chilled. And voila!

Deliver-My-Liver Detox Smoothie

This liver detox smoothie will make your liver leap with joy. Potassium from the banana, the proinflammatory enzymes to fight inflammation from the cucumbers, quercetin in the red apples can help boost and fortify your immune system. Parsley can help control your blood pressure (scientists have labeled it a chemo-protective food). Cayenne pepper can help you lose weight and burn fat, and the grapefruit boosts metabolism!

   1/2 cucumber
   1 carrot
   1/2 grapefruit, peeled
   2 springs of parsley
   Dash of cayenne pepper
   Dash of turmeric
   1 garlic clove (optional)
   1 glass of water

This a delicious, easy drink to make. Add all ingredients into the blender and voila! If this isn't sweet enough for you, add 1 cored red apple. And voila!

Happy-Skin Smoothie

Try something different: freeze 1/2 cup of pure pumpkin (not pumpkin pie mix) in an ice cube tray.

   1/2 cup of ice-cubed pure pumpkin
   7 oz of So Delicious Greek-style coconut milk yogurt
   1/2 cup of vita coconut water
   2 tablespoons of flaxseed meal
   1/2 teaspoon pumpkin spice pie mix

This a delicious, easy drink to make. Add all ingredients into the blender and voila! Your skin, thyroid, and body will thank you. And voila!

Green "Thank the Goddess" Smoothie

1 cup cucumber chunks, peeled
1/2 avocado, peeled and cut into chunks
1 large kiwi, peeled and cut into chunks
1/2 cup fresh OJ
1/4 cup of fresh mint leaves
1 cup of romaine lettuce
4 pitted, dried apricots
5 ice cubes

This a delicious, easy drink to make. Add all ingredients into the blender and voila! If it's too thick, add some more freshly squeezed OJ.

Gingered Cantaloupe Smoothie

2 cups of cantaloupe, cut up
6 oz of Almond Dream plain yogurt
1/2 teaspoon grated fresh ginger
2 springs of fresh parsley
2 stalks of celery
1 cup of water or unsweetened almond milk
5 ice cubes

This a delicious, easy drink to make. Add all ingredients into the blender and voila!

High-C Smoothie

2 celery stalks
1 kiwi, peeled and cut up
2 springs of parsley
1 cup of freshly squeezed OJ
2 tablespoons flaxseed meal

This a delicious, easy drink to make. Add all ingredients into the blender and voila!

Cherry-Pineapple Surprise Smoothie

1 cup organic cherries, frozen
1 cup, chunks pineapple, frozen
1 cup fresh orange juice
1/2 medium bananas
7 oz of So Delicious Greek-style coconut milk yogurt
2 tablespoon flaxseed meal

This a delicious, easy drink to make. Add all ingredients into the blender and voila!

Happy-Colon smoothie

1 cup pumpkin puree
1 tablespoon raw honey
1/2 of a peeled grapefruit
1 cup unsweetened almond milk
2 tablespoon flaxseed meal
1/2 inch fresh raw ginger
1/2 teaspoon cinnamon, nutmeg and turmeric

This a delicious, easy drink to make. Add all ingredients into the blender and voila!

Tropical Coconut Smoothie

1 1/2 coconut water
2 cups frozen pineapple chunks
2 medium bananas
2 cups freshly squeezed orange juice
2 tablespoons flaxseed meal

This a delicious, easy drink to make. Add all ingredients into the blender and voila!

Blueberry Booster Smoothie

1 cup blueberries
1 medium banana, peeled
1 cucumber, peeled and cut up
1 cup of filtered water
1 tablespoon chia seeds

This a delicious, easy drink to make. Add all ingredients into the blender and voila!

Anti-inflammatory Smoothie

1/2 cup frozen pineapple chunks
1 cucumber, peeled and cut up
2 stalks of celery
1 lime, peeled and cut up in wedges
2 springs of fresh parsley
1 cup of coconut water

This a delicious, easy drink to make. Add all ingredients into the blender and voila!

Oatmeal Smoothie

1/2 cup frozen raspberries
7 oz of So Delicious Greek-style coconut milk yogurt
1 banana
1/2 cup old-fashioned, gluten-free, rolled oats
1 tablespoon raw honey
1 cup coconut water
1 cup of ice
2 tablespoons of grounded flaxseed

This a delicious, easy drink to make. Add all ingredients into the blender and voila!

Apple Pie Smoothie

1 large sweet apple, peeled and sliced
1 cup organic romaine lettuce leaves
1/2 banana, peeled
1 teaspoon vanilla extract
1 teaspoon ground cinnamon
1/4 cup raw almonds
1 tablespoon coconut flakes
1 cup coconut milk
1/2 cup ice, optional

This a delicious, easy drink to make. Add all ingredients into the blender. It might take a bit to get the romaine and almonds blended. Top with additional cinnamon if you want an extra kick of flavor and voila!

Skin-Tactic Water

8 glasses water
1 teaspoon grated ginger root (optional)
1 medium-sized cucumber, peeled and cut into slices
1 medium-sized lemon cut into slices
12 fresh mint leaves

Mix all the ingredients in a large pitcher; leave them overnight. Drink all the next day. Voila!

Anti-inflammatory Tonic Recipe

2 cups coconut water (or filtered water)
2 tablespoon grated fresh turmeric—about a 2-inch piece (or 1/2 to 1 tsp. dried turmeric powder)
1 tablespoon grated fresh ginger—about a 1-inch piece
Juice from 1 lemon or orange
1 medium carrot
1 tablespoon raw honey or real maple syrup

Pinch of black pepper
Optional: a pinch of cayenne or cinnamon

This a delicious, easy drink to make. Add all ingredients into the blender and voila!

Breakfast Juice Tonic

Handful of cranberries (1/2 cup)
1 organic carrots
1 organic cucumber
1 organic celery sticks
1 peeled lemon
1 organic granny smith apple
1/2 inch fresh ginger, peeled
1 spring of parsley

Cut to fit in your juicer. Drink and enjoy. Voila!

Golden Milk Health Benefits

It has anti-inflammatory properties and is antibacterial. It's loaded in antioxidants, helps fight infections, improve cognitive ability, helps lubricate the joints, purifies the blood, balance blood sugar, promotes weight loss, and even clear the skin.

1/8 tsp. turmeric
Dash of pepper
Dash of nutmeg or Ceylon cinnamon
1/4 teaspoon of baking soda
1/2 cup water
1 cup coconut milk
Raw, organic honey to taste

Boil water and turmeric for about eight minutes as the turmeric has to be fully cooked. In a separate pot, bring the milk to a boil and remove from heat. Combine the two mixtures and add honey to taste. I would also recommend adding a little nutmeg since it also offers so many amazing healing benefits.

LEMON, GINGER, AND TURMERIC TEA

This is an amazing morning go-to drink. It's healing, energizing, and hydrating. Turmeric is an antioxidant, cancer preventive, anti-inflammatory, and aids in liver protection. Lemon does a fabulous job with alkalinizing the body, aiding in digestion, and boosting your immune system. Ginger is anti-inflammatory, boosts your immune system, lowers blood sugar, lowers cholesterol levels, cancer fighter, improves brain function, prevents cold and flu, and improves heart health. Cloves reduces inflammation, has antiviral and antibacterial properties, improves digestion, aids in relieving sore throat, is a natural painkiller, helps with insomnia, and aids in healthier teeth and gums. Cayenne pepper is a pain reliever, appetite suppressant, helps reduce blood sugar levels, helps remove toxins from the blood, and improves blood circulation.

Word of caution: pregnant women are advised to control consumption since it could stimulate the uterus.

1 whole lemon, sliced
1 tablespoon ginger, minced
2 cloves

1/8 teaspoon turmeric
2 1/2 cups boiling water
Pinch of cayenne

Place the lemon slices, ginger, cloves, and turmeric in a teapot. Pour your boiling water in your teapot. Allow to steep for 30 minutes. Strain over your cup. Just before serving, add a dash of cayenne pepper. If you feel a sore throat coming on, add 2 teaspoons of raw honey. Honey is a natural cough suppressant, has antibacterial properties, and will help reduce swelling and discomfort. If you want it creamy, you can always add coconut milk or almond milk.

The 5 to Stay Alive

This wonderful tonic can be used more than just as a heart health protocol; it's been proven to reduce cholesterol, heal hemorrhoids, clear out arteries for your heart, reduce blood pressure, stop colds in their tracks, ease constipation, heal ulcers, promote weight loss, treats respiratory issues, and you can even put it on a cotton swab and treat acne and pimples. This hasn't been proven, but I also have a theory that I jokingly say, "It repels vampires and unwanted friends who get to close in your personal space."

I've seen various different ways to make it. This is how I make it. Put 3 tablespoons in a glass of water on an empty stomach daily. Garlic, ginger, and even lemon can interact with certain medications. Please check with your health care provider to make sure that you won't have any adverse medication reactions if you plan on taking this as a drink with other medications.

10 gloves of garlic
1 cup of raw honey
1 cup of organic apple cider vinegar
2-inch piece of fresh ginger, peeled
2 lemons, washed and cut

Blend, strain, and store in a mason jar in the refrigeration.

The Morning-After Drink

Not everyone can stomach raw garlic or organic apple cider vinegar. It's just not for everyone. I personally love it. If you are among many others who want to lower their blood pressure but can't drink the 5 to Stay Alive mix, here is a "easier on your taste buds" alternative to help lower your blood pressure. Ceylon cinnamon can help improve glucose and lipid levels, reduce blood sugar levels, lower cholesterol, support healthy blood clotting, and boost memory and protect the brain. Organic apple cider vinegar lowers blood sugar, lowers cholesterol, aids in weight loss, relieves sore throat, and is an energy booster. Fresh lemon is blood purifier, blood sugar balancer, aids in detoxifying, weight loss, insomnia, asthma, and cough and cold. Raw honey has nutritional benefits, promotes the growth of good bacteria in the gut, helps fight insomnia, helps with pollen allergies, and reduces homocysteine levels to maintain a healthy heart. Please check with your health care provider to make sure that you won't have any adverse medication reactions if you plan on taking this as a drink with other medications. Although everything is natural, some natural foods do have adverse reactions when combined with daily medication. Please be aware of your daily medication and if anything you eat or drink will have an adverse reaction when combined.

> 1 teaspoon of Ceylon cinnamon
> 2 tablespoons of organic apple cider vinegar
> Juice of 1 fresh lemon
> 1 tablespoon of raw honey
> 16 oz of filtered water

> Blend until smooth and drink!

Red Onion Tea

What a true gift from nature. Onions are natural fat blockers, promotes a smoother bowel movement, helps relieve common cold, ease asthma, fights bacterial infections, fights respiratory problems and angina, reduces appetite, treats anemia, helps with insomnia, boosts your sex drive, is a cancer fighter, a blood thinner, and relieves the common cold-related cough. Onions have antibacterial and antifungal properties. Onions also contain calcium, magnesium, sodium, potassium, selenium, phosphorus, and they are a good source of vitamin C, vitamin B6, and dietary fiber! The incredible, edible onion.

1 cup of water
1 onion, cut in quarters

Blend, strain and drink.

If you are having problems with your asthma, you can also add 1 tablespoon of raw honey, 1/8 teaspoon of black pepper to a quarter cup of your onion juice. It can help ease your symptoms, but please make sure you follow all your necessary precautions. This isn't to replace what you normally do when you have an asthma attack. Always check with your health care provider before starting a new regime.

SOUPS, SALADS
AND SIDES

It's best to make your own soups to stay away from canned soups to avoid the BPA, aluminum leaks, and preservatives. If you must get prepackaged soups or broths, find those in paper containers. Read the labels and try to avoid MSG, preservatives, and ingredients you can't even pronounce. I will show you how salads can be fresh and never boring along with some simple side recipes to add to any of your meals. Remember: you're either fighting or feeding disease in your body.

Tuna Pasta Salad with Balsamic Vinaigrette

    1 12-ounce box tricolor gluten-free rotini pasta, cooked al dente,
        rinsed in cold water and drained
    1 4-ounce or 5-ounce paper-packed tuna, flaked
    1 cup grape tomatoes, halved
    1/4 cup sliced black olives
    1/2 cup diced fresh zucchini
    3 tablespoons chopped sun-dried tomatoes
    1/4 cup chopped red onion
    1/4 cup crumbled goat cheese
    1 tablespoons Greek seasoning (or more to taste)

For the dressing:

1/4 cup extra-virgin olive oil
1/4 cup white balsamic dressing
1 tablespoon Dijon mustard
1 clove garlic, minced

In large bowl, combine all the salad ingredients. In a mason jar with lid, combine all the dressing ingredients; seal the lid and give a good shake. Pour dressing over the salad and mix to combine. Store in refrigerator for 30 minutes before serving to allow flavors to blend.

Creamy White-Bean-and-Roasted-Mushroom Soup

16 oz. white button mushrooms, chopped
2 large sweet onions, quartered
3 garlic cloves, minced
2 tablespoons olive oil
1 1/2 teaspoon Celtic sea salt, divided
1 1/2 teaspoon pepper, divided
10 fresh sage leaves
10 stems + 1 tablespoon leaves of fresh thyme, divided
48 oz. vegetable broth
3 15-ounce cans organic navy beans, great northern
    or cannellini beans, rinsed and drained

Preheat oven to 450°F. Toss mushrooms, garlic and onion in olive oil, 1 teaspoon salt, and 1 teaspoon pepper spread on baking sheet. Add sage leaves and stems of thyme. Roast in 450°F oven for 10 minutes; toss and roast for additional 15 minutes.

While vegetables are roasting, add broth, beans, 1/2 teaspoon salt, 1/2 teaspoon pepper, and 1 tablespoon fresh thyme leaves to a dutch oven over medium heat and simmer. Once vegetables are done roasting, remove the mushrooms to use as a topping for your soup.

Blend 2 cups of the white beans and 1 cup of broth with the roasted onions, garlic, and herbs. Cover and blend until smooth.

Add pureed bean mixture back to your pot, whisking in until smooth. After you place your soup in your bowl, top with the roasted mushrooms.

White Bean and Butternut Squash Soup

> 3 tablespoon olive oil
> 3 cloves garlic, peeled and minced
> 3 cups butternut squash, peeled, seeded, and cubed
> 1 organic yellow squash, cubed
> 1 can organic navy beans, great northern or cannellini beans, rinsed and drained
> 1 can organic Italian tomatoes, roughly chopped
> 1/2 cup fresh basil and parsley leaves, chopped
> 4 cups vegan, gluten-free broth
> Salt and pepper to taste
> Gluten-free pasta, cooked (optional)

In a dutch oven pot, heat olive oil under medium heat; add garlic and sauté until golden, 3–4 minutes. Add butternut squash and sauté until tender, about 6–8 minutes. Next, add the yellow squash, broth, tomatoes, beans, herbs, and salt and pepper. Turn your heat down to low and simmer for about 20 minutes until squash is tender and broth has reduced some, stirring occasionally. Place your cooked pasta in bowls and top with your stew.

Vegetable Chicken Soup

You can make this without the chicken and make it a vegan soup!

> 2 tablespoons olive oil
> 1 pound boneless, skinless chicken breast, cut into bites-size pieces
> 2 cloves garlic, minced
> 1 onion, chopped
> 4 cups low-sodium chicken broth
> 2 cups of green beans
> 1 1/2 cups frozen corn
> 1 red bell pepper, chopped
> 1 celery, chopped
> 1 small zucchini, quartered lengthwise and sliced
> 1/4 teaspoon salt
> 1/2 teaspoon freshly ground pepper

2 tablespoons chopped fresh parsley
2 can of roasted tomatoes with juice (optional)

Heat the oil in a large dutch oven over medium-high heat. Add the chicken; cook until lightly browned. Add the garlic, red bell pepper, and onion. Cook onion, red bell pepper, and garlic until fragrant. Add the rest of the ingredients. Bring to a boil. Reduce the heat to low, cover, and simmer for 30 minutes. Add the 2 tablespoon of fresh parsley.

Sautéed White Beans and Brown Rice

2 tablespoons coconut oil
1/2 white or yellow onion, finely chopped
1/2 a red bell pepper, chopped
1 stalk of celery, chopped
Kosher salt
1 clove garlic, minced
1 teaspoon ground cumin
1/2 cup white wine
1 1/2 cups cooked navy beans, great northern or cannellini beans
2 tablespoons chopped fresh oregano leaves (or 2 teaspoons dried)
Freshly ground black pepper
2 cups of cooked brown rice

In a cast-iron skillet, over medium heat, add the oil. Sauté the onion, bell pepper, and celery until soft, about 5 minutes. Add the garlic and cumin and cook additional 2 minutes. Raise the heat and add the white wine. Cook until the wine has reduced by half. Stir in the beans and oregano and season with salt and pepper to taste. Cook gently for 15 minutes. Transfer to a serving bowl and serve.

Greek Salad with Chickpeas and Sardines

3 tablespoons lemon juice
2 tablespoons extra-virgin olive oil
1 clove garlic, minced
2 teaspoons dried oregano
1/2 teaspoon freshly ground pepper

3 medium tomatoes, cut into large chunks
1 large English cucumber, cut into large chunks
1 15-ounce can chickpeas, rinsed
1/3 cup crumbled goat cheese
1/4 cup thinly sliced red onion
2 tablespoons sliced Kalamata olives
2 4-ounce cans sardines with bones,
      packed in olive oil or water, drained

Whisk lemon juice, oil, garlic, oregano, and pepper in a large bowl until well combined. Add tomatoes, cucumber, chickpeas, feta, onion, and olives. Toss to combine. Place your salad on plates and top with sardines. Don't worry about the bones in the sardines. You can eat them. They are not hard. They crumble when you bite into them and you can even mash them into a paste.

Sweet Corn Chowder with Hot-Smoked Salmon

1 tablespoon butter
2 cups chopped onion
1 1/2 cups cubed peeled baking potato
3 cups fat-free, less-sodium chicken broth
1 1/2 cups fresh corn kernels
1 15-ounce can no-salt-added cream-style corn
1/4 teaspoon freshly ground black pepper
1/8 teaspoon ground red pepper
2 4.5-ounce packages hot-smoked salmon, flaked
4 teaspoons chopped fresh chives

Melt butter in a cast-iron skillet over medium heat. Add onion; sauté for 4 minutes. Add potato and broth; bring to a boil. Reduce heat and simmer for 10 minutes until the potatoes are tender. Add corn kernels and cream-style corn; cook for 5 minutes. Stir in peppers. Ladle 1 1/4 cups chowder into bowls. Top with your bowls with the salmon and add chives for a nice garnish.

Spicy Tuna Quinoa Salad

  1/2 onion, diced
  1/2 red and 1/2 yellow bell pepper, diced
  1 tablespoon coconut oil or olive oil
  1 tablespoon of crushed red pepper
  1 cup of cooked quinoa in vegetable broth instead of water
  1/4 cup of cherry tomatoes, halved
  1/4 cup black olives, chopped
  1 2.6-ounce pack of (single-serve, ready-to-eat)
      albacore tuna in water

In a cast-iron skillet, sauté onions and peppers in the oil until soft over medium heat. Add the crushed red pepper. Mix the quinoa, onion mixture, cherry tomatoes, olives, and tuna together. Reduce your heat to low and cook additional 5 minutes. Once cooked, place in bowl and chow down!

Tuna and Chickpea Salad

  2 15-ounce cans chickpeas, drained and rinsed
  1 12-ounce can chunk light tuna packed in water, drained
  2 cups cherry tomatoes, halved (quartered if large)
  1/2 cup pitted black olives, chopped
  1 shallot, finely chopped
  1/4 cup finely chopped fresh parsley
  3 tablespoons olive oil
  3 tablespoons lemon juice
  Celtic sea salt and pepper

Lay down a bed of Romaine lettuce. In a large bowl, combine beans, tuna, tomatoes, olives, shallot and parsley. Drizzle oil and lemon juice over mixture. Toss well, season with salt and pepper, and serve over greens.

Egg Salad

12 hard-boiled egg whites with only of the 6 yolks
1 peeled avocado
2 celery stalks, diced small
1/4 cup freshly diced red onion
Salt and pepper

Diced up the eggs and avocado with a fork. Add everything else and mix well. Don't be alarmed that it is greenish in color. The avocado gives it a creamy flavor. Eat the egg salad on gluten-free bread or place in a large romaine lettuce leave and have an egg salad roll-up.

Black Bean Salad

3 cups black beans, cooked and drained
2 cups frozen corn, cooked and drained
2 sweet red or orange bell peppers, cut into pieces
1/2 cup red onion, minced
1/2 cup fresh cilantro, chopped
1/2 cup parsley, chopped
1 teaspoon chili peppers, crushed
3 cloves garlic, crushed
1/2 cup lime juice
1/2 cup EVOO
2 teaspoon cumin
1 teaspoon salt

Combine beans, corn, onions, red peppers, cilantro, parsley, chili peppers. Mix garlic, lime juice, oil, cumin, and salt. You can toss this with some mixed greens.

Greens with Vinaigrette

6 cups romaine lettuce, torn
1/3 cup olive oil
1/4 cup honey
2 teaspoons white wine vinegar or Bragg's Apple Cider Vinegar

1 1/2 teaspoons lemon juice
1/2 teaspoon dry mustard
2 garlic cloves, minced
1 drop hot pepper sauce
Pinch of sugar
Salt and pepper to taste

Place your salad mix in a large bowl. Combine the remaining ingredients in a mason jar with a lid and shake until well combined. Pour your vinaigrette over salad and toss gently

Shoepeg Corn Salad

16 ounces frozen white corn, thawed
1/2 cup red bell or orange or yellow pepper, diced
1 cup onion, diced
2 stalks celery, diced
1/2 cup extra-virgin olive oil
1/2 cup Bragg's Apple Cider Vinegar
1 teaspoon salt
1/2 teaspoon black pepper

Combine everything in a bowl. Mix well to combine.

Tomato and Lentil Soup

2 tablespoons olive oil
1 onion, chopped
2 carrots, chopped
3 cups water
3/4 cup lentils (I used brown lentils, but I
    imagine any type would work)
1 vegetable bouillon cube
14 oz canned chopped tomatoes
2 tablespoons tomato paste, tomato sauce, or ketchup, in a pinch
Paprika and garlic powder, to taste
Salt and pepper, to taste

In a large dutch oven, sauté onions and carrots in olive oil until they begin to soften. Add water and lentils. Simmer over medium heat for about 15 minutes or until lentils begin to soften. Add canned tomatoes, bouillon cube, and tomato paste. Simmer for an additional 10 minutes until lentils are completely soft. You can use an immersion blender to puree the soup or in batches blend.

Chunky Tomato, Roasted Red Bell Pepper, and Quinoa Soup

1/2 cup quinoa
3 tablespoons olive oil
1 large onion, minced
2 stalks celery, chopped
3 cloves garlic, minced
1 tablespoon smoked paprika
Celtic sea salt or Himalayan pink salt
Pepper
1 yellow pepper, diced
1 jar of roasted red peppers, drained and diced
1 can 15-ounce low-sodium diced tomatoes
2 cans 15-ounce low-sodium chickpeas, rinsed
2 cups low-sodium vegetable broth
2 tablespoons red wine vinegar

Rinse the quinoa of needed until water for 5 minutes with a mesh strainer. Cook the quinoa according to package directions.

Meanwhile, heat the oil in a dutch oven or large, heavy-bottomed pot. Sauté the onion, celery, yellow bell pepper, and garlic, stirring occasionally. Cook until onions are translucent, about 5 minutes.

Add the diced roasted red bell peppers, paprika, and 1/4 teaspoon each of salt and pepper, and cook, stirring for 2 minutes. Add the peppers and cook, stirring occasionally for 5 minutes.

Add the chickpeas, broth, and 1 cup water and bring to a boil. Reduce heat and simmer until the vegetables are tender, 5 to 8 minutes. Stir in the vinegar and cooked quinoa. Ladle in to bowls and eat!

Roasted Butternut Squash Soup

> 1 butternut squash, peeled, seeded and cubed into 3/4-inch pieces
> (approx. 4 cups)
> 3 garlic cloves, peeled and chopped
> 1/2 sweet onion, peeled and halved
> 1 tablespoon olive or coconut oil
> 1/2 teaspoon Celtic sea salt
> 2 1/2 low-sodium vegetable broth

Preheat oven to 400 degrees. Toss your prepared vegetables with olive oil on place them on a large cast-iron skillet for roasting. Stir a few times to make sure squash is fork-tender and roast for 40 minutes. Remove any onion or garlic that seemed to be overroasted and set aside. After you've roasted them for 40 minutes, allow them to cool for 10 to 15 min. Remove any garlic or onions that have overroasted.

Place your roasted mixture in a blender or a food processor and blend until creamy. In large pot, place blended mix and broth and salt. Cook on medium low until heated, adding more liquid as needed and taste for seasoning.

I like topping my soup with raw pumpkin seeds and a dash of cayenne pepper for some heat.

Roasted Red Pepper and Tomato Soup

> 10 medium-sized vine-ripened tomatoes, quartered
> 1 small onion, quartered
> 4 cloves of garlic
> 2 red bell peppers, seeds removed and quartered
> 1/4 teaspoon thyme
> A few sprigs of rosemary
> Celtic sea salt and ground black pepper
> 1 tablespoon olive oil
> 1 cup low-sodium vegetable broth
> 3 tablespoons tomato paste
> A handful of fresh basil leaves

Preheat oven to 350° F. Toss your prepared vegetables including your garlic and rosemary with olive oil and place them in a cast-iron skillet. Sprinkle with thyme, sea salt, and freshly ground black pepper and mix well to combine.

Roast veggies for 45–50 minutes or until tender and lightly browned. Blend your roasted mix in a blender or a food processor until the soup is thick and creamy. In large pot, place blended mix. If it's too thick, you might want to add a little bit more veggie broth. Cook on medium low until heated, adding more liquid as needed and taste for seasoning.

Mexican Lentil Tortilla Soup

2 tablespoons extra-virgin olive oil
1 cup diced yellow onion
1/2 cup diced celery
1 cup diced carrots
2 cloves garlic, minced
1/2 cup lentils rinsed
6 cups vegetable broth
1 14-ounce jar crushed tomatoes
1/2 jalapeno pepper, seeded and minced
1/2 teaspoon ground cumin
1/2 teaspoon ground coriander
1/2 teaspoon sea salt, more as needed
1/4 teaspoon pepper, more as needed
1/4 cup chopped fresh cilantro
3 corn tortillas, cut in 1/2-inch-wide pieces

Optional Toppings:

Sliced avocado
Goat cheese
A squeeze of fresh lime

In a dutch oven, over medium heat, add your olive oil. Make sure pan is coated. Place your onion, celery, and carrots and cook until tender, 8–10 minutes. Add the garlic and cook 1 minute. Add the lentils, vegetable broth, tomatoes, jalapeno, cumin, coriander, salt, pepper, cilantro, and tortilla strips. Bring to a boil and turn down the heat to a simmer. Cook for 20–25 minutes. Once completely done, using ladles, place your soup in a bowl and top with the sliced avocado, goat cheese, and a squeeze of lime for an extra zing!

Black Bean Soup

    1 tablespoon olive oil
    1 medium onion, diced
    1 1/2 tablespoons chili powder
    1 1/2 tablespoons oregano
    1 teaspoon cumin
    1/2 teaspoon salt
    1/2 teaspoon black pepper
    4 cloves garlic, minced
    3 15-ounce cans black beans, drained but not rinsed
    3 cups water
    2 bay leaves
    1/2 cup fresh cilantro, roughly chopped

In a dutch oven, heat oil over medium heat. Add the onion; cook until translucent, about 5 minutes. Mix in the spices, salt, pepper, and garlic and cook for another 1–2 minutes until fragrant. Add your black beans; mix well to combine with the spices and onions and cook for 1–2 minutes more. Next, add the water and bay leaves. Bring your soup to a boil. Once it starts to boil, reduce the heat and simmer uncovered for 25 minutes.

Before you start to blend, don't forget those bay leaves! You can use an immersion blender, food processor, or blender to puree the soup until smooth, but you still want some chunks and texture in the soup. Ladle into bowls. Top with chopped cilantro, avocado, and scallions.

White Bean Salad Recipe

    1 14.5-ounce can navy beans, cannellini beans or great northern, drained and rinsed
    2 tablespoons red onion, chopped
    2 teaspoons red wine vinegar

2 tablespoons extra-virgin olive oil
1/2 teaspoon dry herbs (rosemary, tarragon, and thyme)
Salt and freshly ground pepper to taste

Mix all your ingredients in a bowl and let it marinate in the fridge for a few hours.

White Bean and Tuna Salad

1 cup of red onions, chopped
1 cup of red bell pepper, chopped
2 tablespoon of organic apple cider vinegar
2 tablespoons of extra-virgin olive oil
2 6-ounce cans of tuna packed in water
2 15-ounce cans of cannellini or great northern
    white beans, rinsed and drained
A few splashes of Tabasco sauce
1/2 teaspoon freshly ground black pepper

Drain the water from the tuna and put the tuna into a large mixing bowl. Add the beans to the tuna and gently stir to combine. Add the rest of the ingredients and mix. Allow it to marinate in the fridge for at least 30 minutes for all the flavors to combine. You can eat this over a bed of salad mix and add some diced tomatoes on top.

Cucumber-Tomato Salad

3 cups of cucumbers, peeled and sliced
3 roma tomatoes, diced
1/4 cup red onion, chopped red onion
1/4 cup chopped fresh basil
1/4 cup extra-virgin olive oil
1/2 cup organic apple cider vinegar
1/2 teaspoon dill weed
Salt and pepper, to taste

Place all the ingredients in large bowl. Mix well to combine. You can eat this plain or on a bed of mixed salad greens.

Simple Squash Salad

1 medium zucchini, washed and sliced
1 medium yellow squash, washed and sliced
Pinch of Himalayan sea salt
1 tablespoon extra-virgin olive oil
1 teaspoon fresh lemon juice
1 garlic clove, minced
1/4 teaspoon freshly ground black pepper

Slice the zucchini and squash into bite-size pieces. Place zucchini and squash in a medium bowl and toss with salt. In a bowl, whisk together extra-virgin olive oil, fresh lemon juice, and minced garlic clove. Pour dressing over squash. Allow to marinate for 30 minutes.

Squash, Chickpea, and Red Lentil Soup

2 cans of chickpeas, drained and rinsed
2 1/2 butternut squash, peeled, seeded and cut into 1-inch cubes
2 large carrots, peeled and cut into bite size pieces
1 large onion, chopped
1 cup red lentils
4 cups vegetable broth
2 tablespoons tomato paste
1 tablespoon minced peeled fresh ginger
1 1/2 teaspoons ground cumin
1 teaspoon salt
1/4 teaspoon freshly ground pepper
1/4 cup lime juice
1/4 cup packed fresh cilantro leaves, chopped

In a dutch oven, heat oil over medium heat. Add the onion; cook until translucent, about 5 minutes. Stir in the remaining ingredients: chickpeas, squash, carrots, lentils, broth, tomato paste, ginger, cumin, salt. Mix well to combine. You want your soup to simmer as it cooks, stirring frequently to avoid sticking. Cover and allow to cook for 45 minutes. Ladle into bowls and squeeze fresh lime on your soup and garnish with cilantro.

Mediterranean Tuna Antipasto Salad

1 15-ounce can chickpeas, drained and rinsed
2 5- to 6-ounce cans water-packed albacore
    tuna, drained and flaked
1 large red bell pepper, diced
1/2 cup red onion, diced
1/2 cup chopped fresh parsley, divided
4 teaspoons capers, rinsed
1 1/2 teaspoons finely chopped fresh rosemary
1/2 cup lemon juice, divided
4 tablespoons extra-virgin olive oil, divided
Freshly ground pepper, to taste
1/4 teaspoon salt
8 cups mixed salad greens

Combine beans, tuna, bell pepper, onion, parsley, capers, rosemary, 1/4 cup lemon juice, and 2 tablespoons oil in a medium bowl. Season with freshly ground pepper. In a large bowl, mix the remaining 1/4 cup lemon juice, 2 tablespoons oil, and salt. Add your salad mix; toss to coat. Place your tossed salad mix onto plates and top each with the tuna salad.

Quinoa, Chickpea, and Avocado Salad

1 cup grape tomatoes, diced
15 oz. can garbanzo beans, rinsed and drained
1 cup cooked quinoa
2 tbsp. red onion, minced
1 cup diced cucumber
4 oz. diced avocado (1 medium hass)
2 tbsp. cilantro, minced
1 1/2 limes, juiced
Himalayan sea salt and fresh pepper, to taste

Combine all the ingredients season with salt and pepper to taste. You can eat this over a fresh salad mix. Reminder: if not eaten immediately, the avocado will turn brown quickly and the cucumber will sweat and make your salad soggy. So if you plan on eating this later, wait until you are ready to serve to add the freshly diced avocado and diced cucumber.

Brown Rice with Tomato and Avocado Salad

1 cup cooked brown rice, cooled to room temp
5 cherry tomatoes, diced
1 avocado, diced
1 garlic cloves, minced
1 tablespoon olive oil
1 lemon, squeezed

Cook brown rice as directed and set let cool. Mix all ingredients together. Season to taste and serve.

Grilled Greek-style Grilled Asparagus Salad with Tomatoes and Goat Cheese

1 bunch asparagus, washed and trimmed
2 tablespoons extra-virgin olive oil
Salt and freshly ground black pepper
1 pint cherry tomatoes, cut in half
1/2 cup sliced red onion
1/2 cup goat cheese

For the vinaigrette:

3 tablespoons extra-virgin olive oil
2 tablespoons red wine vinegar
1 teaspoon Dijon mustard
1/2 teaspoon dried rosemary
1/2 teaspoon salt
1/4 teaspoon freshly ground black pepper

Preheat grill to high heat. Lightly coat the asparagus spears with olive oil. Season with salt and pepper to taste. Grill over high heat for 2 to 3 minutes, or to desired tenderness. Place the asparagus, red onion, and cherry tomatoes in a large mixing bowl. To prepare the vinaigrette, combine all ingredients and mix until well blended.

Pour the vinaigrette over the vegetables and gently toss to combine. Add the goat's cheese and very carefully stir to combine. Let sit for at least 30 minutes before serving.

Three-Bean Salad

1 15-ounce can cannellini beans, drained and rinsed
1 15-ounce can chickpeas, drained and rinsed
1 15-ounce can kidney beans, drained and rinsed
2 celery stalks, finely chopped
1/2 red onion, finely chopped
1 tablespoons dried rosemary
3 tablespoons red wine vinegar
1/4 cup extra-virgin olive oil
Himalayan sea salt and pepper to taste

In a large bowl, mix the cannellini beans, chickpeas, kidney beans, celery, onion, and rosemary. In a small bowl, whisk together the red wine vinegar, oil, salt, and pepper. Pour the vinaigrette over the beans and mix well.

Sautéed Mushrooms, Onions, and Garlic

3 cups of baby mushrooms, cut off ends
1 medium onion, sliced
1 garlic clove, minced
2 tablespoon extra-virgin olive oil
1 tablespoons of Bragg's Liquid Aminos
1/4 cup of white wine

Cut your mushroom stems off and gently wipe off any dirt debris you may find on it. Heat a cast-iron skillet to medium high heat. Add your olive oil. Sautee your onions and garlic for 5 minutes, until softened and fragrant. Keep stirring with a wooden spoon to make sure it doesn't stick. Add you mushrooms and cook for 10 additional minutes. Mix the onion, mushroom, and garlic mixture to combine and stir frequently. Add 1 tablespoon of Bragg's Liquid Aminos. Mix well then add your white wine. Mix well and cook until wine evaporates.

Buttery Baked Spaghetti Squash with Garlic

  1 small spaghetti squash (about 3–4 pounds)
  2 tablespoons nonsoy or nondairy butter
  2 cloves garlic, finely minced
  1/4 cup finely minced parsley
  Himalayan sea salt and pepper to taste

Preheat your oven to 425°F. Wash and cut your squash in half. Scrap out the seeds and discard. Sprinkle extra-virgin olive oil and salt and pepper. Lay scooped side down flat on your baking sheet. Bake your spaghetti squash for 60 minutes. Let squash rest for 10 minutes. After 10 minutes of cooling off, use a fork to scrape the squash to get long, beautiful strands. Heat a cast-iron skillet. Add 2 tablespoons of butter to your pan. Sautee the garlic over medium-low heat. When garlic becomes fragrant, add spaghetti squash. Toss well. Cook for additional 5 minutes.

Savory Balsamic Glazed Carrots

  3 cups baby carrots
  1 tablespoon olive oil
  1 1/2 tablespoons balsamic vinegar
  1 tablespoon brown sugar

Heat oil in a cast-iron skillet over medium-high heat. Sauté carrots in olive oil for about 10 minutes or until soft. Stir in balsamic vinegar and brown sugar; mix well to coat.

Grilled Zucchini

  2 teaspoons extra-virgin olive oil
  1/4 teaspoon Himalayan sea salt
  1/4 teaspoon freshly ground black pepper
  2 medium zucchini, cut into spear-size quarters, lengthwise

Preheat your grill pan over medium-high heat. Combine all ingredients in a bowl and mix well to coat. Lay the zucchini in a single layer on the pan. Grill for 4 minutes, turning after 2 minutes.

Roasted Coconut-Lime-Baked Squash

1 butternut squash peeled, seeds discarded and diced
3 tablespoon of melted coconut oil
Juice and zest from 1 lime juice
2 tablespoon honey

Preheat oven to 425°F. In a large bowl, place your diced squash and mix well with all the ingredients. Place a baking sheet and bake for 30–45 minutes or until squash is fork-tender.

Baby Sweet Peas and Onions

1 pound baby sweet peas, fresh or frozen
1 onion, chopped fine
3 tablespoons nonsoy or nondairy butter
1/2 cup gluten-free, low-sodium chicken stock
Black pepper and Himalayan Sea salt to taste

In a cast-iron skillet, heat the butter to melt and sauté the onions for 3–5 minutes. Next, add the peas and the chicken stock and bring to a rolling boil. Allow to cook and the broth to be reduced by half. Season with salt and pepper.

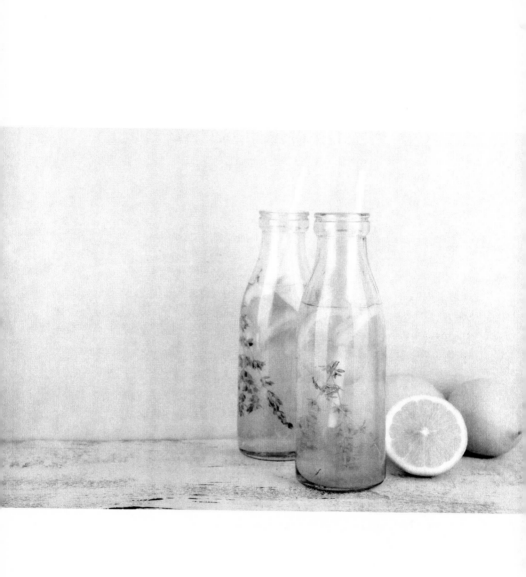

EASY, QUICK, AND HEALTHY HOMEMADE SALAD DRESSINGS

Many over-the-counter salad dressings are filled with trans fats, sugar, preservatives, and artificial ingredients and flavors. Read the labels. You will be shocked to see some words like *calcium disodium EDTA*, *canola oil* (and/or soybean oil), *caramel color, cellulose gum, cornstarch* (or modified cornstarch), *disodium guanylate, disodium inosinate, gum arabic, MSG* (monosodium glutamate), *polysorbate 60, potassium sorbate, sodium* and *calcium caseinates*. You can easily make your own salad dressings with a few ingredients. All it takes is a little extra time. Do you want your salad dressing to come from a lab or your kitchen?

All the vinaigrette recipes can be prepared ahead and refrigerated in a mason jar with a tightly sealed lid up to 1 week.

Honey OACV Dijon Vinaigrette

1/3 cup EVOO
3 tablespoons organic apple cider vinegar
1 tablespoon raw honey
1 tablespoon Dijon mustard
1/4 teaspoon basil
1 small shallot, minced

Pour all the ingredients in a mason jar with a lid and give a good shake to combine. You can season with Himalayan sea salt and freshly ground black pepper. Store in refrigerator.

Dijon Vinaigrette

> 2 garlic gloves, minced
> 1/2 tablespoon Dijon mustard
> 1 teaspoon lemon juice
> 3 tablespoon extra-virgin olive oil

Pour all the ingredients in a mason jar with a lid and give a good shake to combine. You can season with Himalayan sea salt and freshly ground black pepper. Store in refrigerator.

Shallot and Grapefruit Dressing

> 1/2 cup shallot, minced
> 1/4 cup freshly squeezed pink grapefruit juice
> 2 tablespoon fresh cilantro, chopped
> 1/2 cup extra-virgin olive oil

Pour all the ingredients in a mason jar with a lid and give a good shake to combine. You can season with Himalayan sea salt and freshly ground black pepper. Store in refrigerator.

Orange-Balsamic Vinaigrette

> 1/4 cup extra-virgin olive oil
> 1/8 cup freshly squeezed orange
> 1/8 balsamic vinegar
> 1 tablespoon Dijon mustard

Pour all the ingredients in a mason jar with a lid and give a good shake to combine. You can season with Himalayan sea salt and freshly ground black pepper. Store in refrigerator.

Lemony Dijon Vinaigrette

3 tablespoons freshly squeezed lemon juice
1/2 teaspoon Dijon mustard
3/4 cup extra-virgin olive oil

Whisk lemon, Dijon mustard, and EVOO together. Pour all the ingredients in a mason jar with a lid and give a good shake to combine. You can season with Himalayan sea salt and freshly ground black pepper. Store in refrigerator.

Red Wine Vinaigrette

2 tablespoons red wine vinegar
1 teaspoon Dijon mustard (optional)
1 small garlic clove, minced (optional)
1/3 cup extra-virgin olive oil
Coarse salt and ground pepper

Pour all the ingredients in a mason jar with a lid and give a good shake to combine. You can season with Himalayan sea salt and freshly ground black pepper. Store in refrigerator.

Honey-Balsamic Vinaigrette

2 tablespoons balsamic vinegar
1 tablespoon raw honey
1 teaspoon Dijon mustard
1/4 cup extra-virgin olive oil
1 garlic glove, minced
Freshly ground black pepper and Himalayan sea salt to taste

Pour all the ingredients in a mason jar with a lid and give a good shake to combine. You can season with Himalayan sea salt and freshly ground black pepper. Store in refrigerator.

Simple Lemon Vinaigrette

1/2 teaspoon finely grated lemon zest
2 tablespoons freshly squeezed lemon juice
1 teaspoon sugar
1/2 teaspoon Dijon mustard
1/4 teaspoon fine sea salt, or to taste
3 to 4 tablespoons extra-virgin olive oil
Freshly ground black pepper to taste

Pour all the ingredients in a mason jar with a lid and give a good shake to combine. You can season with Himalayan sea salt and freshly ground black pepper. Store in refrigerator.

Basic Vinaigrette

1 cup olive oil
1/4 cup organic apple cider vinegar
1 teaspoon garlic powder
1 teaspoon onion powder
1 teaspoon Celtic sea salt
1/2 teaspoon black pepper

Pour all the ingredients in a mason jar with a lid and give a good shake to combine. You can season with Himalayan sea salt and freshly ground black pepper. Store in refrigerator.

Cucumber–Coconut Milk Ranch Dressing

1 can full-fat coconut milk or coconut cream, refrigerated overnight
1 medium cucumber, peeled, halved lengthwise, seeded, and grated on the large holes of a box grater
2 tablespoons minced shallots
1 garlic clove, minced
2 tablespoons organic apple cider vinegar
3 tablespoons chopped fresh chives
1 1/2 tablespoons chopped fresh parsley

1 1/2 tablespoons chopped fresh basil
1 tablespoon chopped fresh dill
Pinch of cayenne pepper
Freshly ground black pepper and Himalayan Sea salt to taste

Open the can of full-fat coconut milk; scoop cream off the top of the can and add it to a large mason jar, leaving the coconut water within the can.

Add 4 tablespoons of the coconut water into the coconut cream and whisk until smooth (save some of the leftover coconut water; you may need to whisk in an extra tablespoon or two after refrigerating your dressing, depending on your desired thickness).

Add in the shallots, garlic, cucumber, apple cider vinegar, chives, cayenne, parsley, basil, dill, sea salt, and black pepper in the mason jar. Close lid tightly, shake until combined and refrigerate dressing for at least 30 minutes to let the flavors combine together. Store in refrigerator.

Honey-Mustard Vinaigrette

1 clove garlic, minced
1 tablespoon white wine vinegar
1 1/2 teaspoons Dijon mustard (coarse or smooth)
1/2 teaspoon raw honey
1/3 cup extra-virgin olive oil
Freshly ground black pepper and Himalayan sea salt to taste

Pour all the ingredients in a mason jar with a lid and give a good shake to combine. You can season with Himalayan sea salt and freshly ground black pepper. Store in refrigerator.

Basic French Vinaigrette

2 tablespoons finely chopped shallots
2 tablespoons red wine vinegar
2 teaspoons Dijon mustard
6 tablespoons extra-virgin olive oil
Freshly ground black pepper and Himalayan sea salt to taste

Pour all the ingredients in a mason jar with a lid and give a good shake to combine. You can season with Himalayan sea salt and freshly ground black pepper. Store in refrigerator.

Coconut-Ginger Dressing

> 2 tablespoons virgin coconut oil
> 2 tablespoons raw honey
> 2 tablespoons lime juice
> 1/2 teaspoon fresh grated ginger (add more if you like ginger)
> 1/4 teaspoon Himalayan sea salt

Throw the oil in a microwave-safe bowl for a few seconds to melt. Mix the grated ginger, coconut oil, and honey with a wire whisk. Add lime juice and salt. Put the entire mixture in a mason jar, seal with a lid, and give a good shake to combine all ingredients.

Refrigerate any leftovers. Once removed from the refrigerator, you will need to heat it over very low heat or allow to get to room temp—oil will solidify and will need to melt. Shake again and add to salad.

Coconut–Honey Mustard Dressing

> 1/4 cup homemade coconut mayonnaise
> 1/4 cup mustard
> 1/2 cup raw honey
> 1/2 teaspoon Bragg's organic apple cider vinegar

Blend all ingredients together in a small bowl with a wire whisk and drizzle over your favorite salad. Add a zing top your salad with some toasted coconut. Store in refrigerator.

Coconut Mayonnaise

Being Southern, it's no secret that I love mayo! Homemade mayo tastes so much better than store-bought, and it is much healthier because there are no trans fats, and you know exactly what is in your mayonnaise.

> 1 whole egg
> 2 egg yolks

1 tablespoon mustard

1 tablespoon fresh lemon juice

1/2 teaspoon salt

1/4 teaspoon pepper

1/2 cup Virgin Coconut Oil (melted if solid)

1/2 cup virgin olive oil

Place the eggs, mustard, lemon juice, salt, and pepper into a food processor or blender. Blend for a few moments. While the food processor is running on low speed, start adding your oils very slowly. Start out with drops and then work up to about a slow and steady stream. This will take a few minutes. Continue blending until all the oil is gone. Add to a mason jar, seal with lid, and store in refrigerator.

Greek Salad Dressing

1/3 cup extra-virgin olive oil

1/3 cup red wine vinegar

1 teaspoon garlic, minced finely

1 teaspoon Dijon mustard

3/4 teaspoon dried basil

3/4 teaspoon dried oregano

1/2 teaspoon salt

1/2 teaspoon pepper

Pour all the ingredients in a mason jar with a lid and give a good shake to combine. You can season with Himalayan sea salt and freshly ground black pepper. Store in refrigerator.

Homemade Ketchup

1 cup organic tomato paste

1 tablespoon raw organic honey

1 tablespoon raw unfiltered apple cider vinegar

1/4 teaspoon mustard

1/4 teaspoon pink Himalayan sea salt

1/4 cup water

Whisk all ingredients together in a bowl, pour in a mason jar, seal with a lid and enjoy! Store in refrigerator.

Lime-Cilantro Marinade

You can use this marinade with fish, chicken, or shrimp.

Juice of 4 limes
1 small red bell pepper
1 bunch cilantro
7 cloves garlic
1 tablespoon olive oil
A few grinds of fresh black pepper

Blend all ingredients in a blender until extra smooth. You can marinate overnight or a few hours. You can also add this mixture to your raw meat and then freeze.

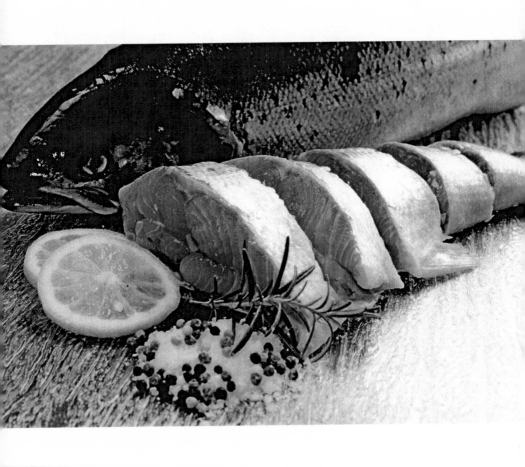

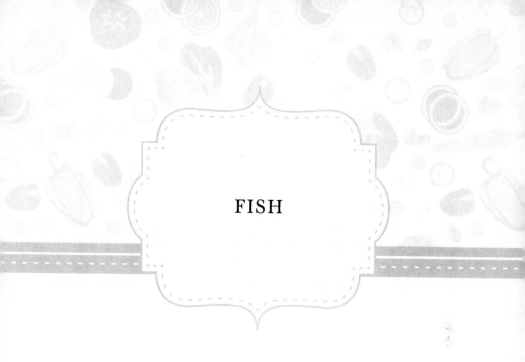

FISH

Did you know?

Salmon contains vitamin D—an essential nutrient that works with calcium to prevent bone loss. Salmon, tuna, and sardines also carry a mega dose of omega-3 fatty acids that keep you healthy. Your body doesn't naturally produce these fatty acids, so you have to get them from food. If you're not into fish, get your vitamin D from cage-free eggs and mushrooms and your omega-3s from walnuts, olive oil, and flaxseed oil. Fish is also a good source of the nutrient selenium, which helps decreases inflammation. Try to eats foods with these "must have feed your body" nutrients daily. Here are seven fish recipes to help decrease inflammation, help with your immunity, lower the risk for heart disease, and supply you with vitamin D and omega-3s for healthier thyroid. Eat more sardines, albacore white tuna, herring, cod, and halibut.

Sweet Corn Chowder with Hot-Smoked Salmon

  1 tablespoon nondairy or nonsoy butter
  2 cups chopped onion
  1 1/2 cups cubed peeled baking potato

3 cups fat-free, less-sodium chicken broth
1 1/2 cups fresh corn kernels
1 15-ounce can no-salt-added cream-style corn
1/4 teaspoon freshly ground black pepper
1/8 teaspoon ground red pepper
2 4.5-ounce packages hot-smoked salmon, flaked
4 teaspoons chopped fresh chives

Melt butter in a large saucepan over medium-high heat. Add onion; sauté for 4 minutes until soft. Add potato and broth; bring to a boil. Reduce heat and simmer for 10 minutes or until potato is tender. Add corn kernels and cream-style corn; cook for 5 minutes. Stir in peppers. Ladle 1 1/4 cups chowder into each of 4 soup bowls. Divide salmon evenly among bowls. Garnish each serving with 1 teaspoon chives.

Salmon Cakes

This is a really super easy way to make salmon patties. Just mix salmon, eggs, onion, and black pepper. Shape into patties, and you're ready to go.

1 14-ounce can salmon, drained and flaked
2 eggs, beaten
1 small onion, diced
1 teaspoon black pepper
3 tablespoon of extra-virgin olive oil or raw coconut oil

Pick through the salmon and remove any bones. In a mixing bowl, beat the eggs and add the diced onion, salmon, and pepper. Mix thoroughly.
Shape into 2-ounce patties; this will make about 7 or 8 patties. In a large cast-iron skillet over medium heat, heat the oil. Fry each patty for about 5 minutes on each side or until crispy and golden brown.

Spicy Fish Taco Bowls

1 tablespoon chili powder
1 tablespoon cumin
1/2 teaspoon cayenne pepper
3–4 salmon filets

1–2 cloves minced garlic
1 cup fresh sweet corn kernels (sliced off the cob is the best)
1 red onion, diced
1 red pepper, diced
1 can black beans, rinsed
2 cups cooked brown rice

You can add a little zip and zing by adding fresh cilantro, avocado, goat's milk cheese, or pico de gallo for topping

Mix the spices together in a small bowl and sprinkle the mixture evenly over both sides of the fish. In a large cast-iron skillet over medium-high heat, heat up a drizzle of olive oil. Add the garlic and sauté for 1–2 minutes. Add the fish to the pan (skin side up; we want a good sear). Cook the fish on each side for several minutes, checking the middle for doneness (fish should be completely white and flake apart easily). Remove fish and set aside. Remove the skin portion on salmon.

Add corn, red peppers, and onions to the pan with no additional oil. Heat over medium heat for several minutes. Do not stir for several minutes; we want it to get a brown/black roasted look on the outside of the mixture. Do this for several minutes (stir, wait, stir, wait) until the peppers and onions are tender-crisp. After this is done, add your black beans and completely heat through.

You can layer this by placing the rice first then the corn-pepper mixture and fish on top in a bowl, or mix everything together in your cast-iron the skillet. Top with any of the toppings listed above for an extra zip and zing!

Teriyaki Salmon with Zucchini

Low-sodium teriyaki sauce
2 6-ounce wild Alaskan salmon fillets
Sesame seeds
2 small zucchini, thinly sliced
4 scallions, chopped
Extra-virgin olive oil or raw coconut oil

Combine 5 tablespoons teriyaki sauce and fish in a zip-top plastic bag. Seal and marinate 20 minutes. Toast sesame seeds in a large cast-iron skillet over medium heat and set aside. Drain fish, discarding marinade. Add fish to the cast-iron skillet and cook 5 minutes. Turn and cook for 5 more minutes over medium-low heat. Remove from skillet and keep warm. Add the zucchini, scallions, and 2 teaspoons oil to skillet. Sauté for 4 minutes or until lightly browned. Stir in 2 tablespoons teriyaki sauce. Sprinkle with sesame seeds and serve with salmon.

Greek Salad with Sardines

    3 tablespoons lemon juice
    2 tablespoons extra-virgin olive oil
    1 clove garlic, minced
    2 teaspoons dried oregano
    1/2 teaspoon freshly ground pepper
    3 medium tomatoes, cut into large chunks
    1 large English cucumber, cut into large chunks
    1 15-ounce can chickpeas, rinsed and drained
    1/3 cup crumbled goat cheese
    1/4 cup thinly sliced red onion
    2 tablespoons sliced Kalamata olives
    2 4-ounce cans sardines with bones, packed in water, drained

Whisk lemon juice, oil, garlic, oregano, and pepper in a large bowl until well combined. Add tomatoes, cucumber, chickpeas, feta, onion, and olives. Mix well to combine. Ladle the salad on plate and top with sardines.

Smoky Artichoke-Sardine Salad

    1/2 cup extra-virgin olive oil
    3 tablespoons sherry vinegar
    1 large shallot, minced
    1 teaspoon Dijon mustard
    3/4 teaspoon smoked paprika
    1/4 teaspoon salt
    1/4 teaspoon freshly ground pepper
    3 cups mixed salad greens
    1/2 cup canned artichoke hearts, rinsed

2 ounces canned sardines
1/4 cup diced red onion

First, place the ingredients for the dressing (vinegar, shallot, mustard, paprika, and salt) in a mason jar with lid shake well to combine. Next, place your salad mix in a bowl and toss with 2 tablespoons of the dressing. (Refrigerate to store the remaining dressing.) Top the greens with artichoke hearts, sardines, and diced red onion.

Quinoa and Tuna Salad

1 cup cooked quinoa
2 cans albacore tuna, drained
1 can petite baby sweet peas, drained and rinsed
2 roma tomatoes, chopped
1/2 cup red bell pepper, diced
1/4 cup red onion, diced
1/2 cup mayonnaise
1 teaspoon garlic, minced
1 teaspoon onion powder
Plenty of salt and pepper to taste

It's so simple! Mix everything in a bowl and serve.

Tuna-Stuffed Peppers

3 sweet bell peppers (red, orange, or yellow)
    sliced in half and deseeded
2 cans of albacore tuna in water, drained
3 tomatoes, peeled and diced
1 tablespoon olive oil
2 cloves garlic, minced
1 onion, diced
1 cup of grumbled goat cheese
1 teaspoon dried thyme leaves, chopped
3 eggs
Salt and freshly ground black pepper

Preheat your oven to 400°F. Slice your peppers in half and remove ribs and seeds. Cut 1/2 of the peppers in small cubes. Heat a large cast-iron skillet over medium-high heat; add olive oil. Add onion, tomatoes, and diced pepper and cook for 1 minute. Add garlic and sauté for 2–3 additional minutes before adding tomato and thyme and cook for another 3 minutes. In a bowl, mix tuna, eggs, and 1/2 cup goat cheese. Mix well. Lay your peppers cut side up in a baking dish and divide the tuna mixture into each pepper. Bake peppers and tuna mixture for 15 minutes. Cover with a foil or parchment pepper to avoid burning the peppers. Remove from oven. Season with Himalayan sea salt, pepper, and goat cheese; cook for 15 more minutes.

Blackened Salmon and Brown Rice

> 2 cups instant brown rice
> 2 1/2 tablespoons paprika
> 3/4 teaspoon cayenne pepper
> 1 teaspoon dried thyme
> 1/2 teaspoon garlic powder
> 1 1/2 teaspoons kosher salt
> 3 1/2 tablespoons Earth Balance butter
> Juice of 1 lemon
> 4 6-ounce salmon fillets, skinned
> 1 11-ounce can corn kernels, drained
> 1/3 cup finely chopped fresh flat-leaf parsley
> 1 lime, cut into wedges

Preheat your oven to 400° F. Cook the rice according to the package directions. Meanwhile, in a small bowl, combine all the spices (paprika, cayenne, thyme, garlic powder, and 1/2 teaspoon of the salt). In a small microwavable bowl melt 2 1/2 tablespoons of the butter. After melted, add the lemon juice and combine the two. Dip each salmon fillet in the lemon-butter mixture and then the spices mixture. Meanwhile, heat a cast-iron skillet over medium-high heat and cook the salmon until blackened, 2 minutes per side. Transfer the pan to the oven for 8 minutes. Mix the corn, parsley, and remaining salt and butter into the rice. Put a bed of rice on a plate. Once the salmon is cooked, lay it on top of the bed of rice and squeeze the juice from the lime wedge over the salmon.

Spaghetti Squash Puttanesca

1 spaghetti squash, cleaned, cut in half, and scraped out of seeds
2 tablespoon olive oil
4–6 anchovies fillets packed in oil, chopped
3–4 garlic cloves, minced
A handful of fresh basil leaves, chopped
14 oz crushed tomatoes
1/3 cup black olives, pitted
Freshly grated parmesan cheese

Clean, cut in half, long way, scrap out seeds and inside of the spaghetti squash. Season with salt, pepper and sprinkle with olive oil. Place in a 400° F oven on a baking pan for 30 minutes. Meanwhile, sauté chopped anchovies in olive oil over low heat while stirring and breaking them up with the wooden spoon for 1–2 minutes; they will start to turn into a paste. Add garlic and continue stirring for 1 minute. Add tomatoes, chopped basil, and olives. Turn the heat up and bring the sauce to a boil. Lower the heat to low and simmer for 6–7 more minutes. Stir occasionally and try to break up big tomatoes chunks with the wooden spoon. Once your spaghetti squash has finished cooking, pull out of oven and allow to cool. Once cooled, scrap the squash with a fork; the flesh will look like strings of spaghetti. Place on your plates; top with your sauce and freshly grated parmesan cheese.

Lemon-Garlic Sardine-Quinoa Fettuccine

8 ounces quinoa fettuccine pasta
4 tablespoons extra-virgin olive oil, divided
4 cloves garlic, minced
1/4 cup lemon juice
1 teaspoon freshly ground pepper
1/2 teaspoon salt
2 3- to 4-ounce cans boneless, skinless sardines,
    preferably in tomato sauce, flaked

1/2 cup chopped fresh parsley
1/4 cup finely shredded parmesan cheese

Bring a large pot of water to a boil. Cook pasta until just tender, 8 to 10 minutes or according to package directions. Drain. Meanwhile, heat 2 tablespoons oil in a cast-iron skillet over medium heat. Add garlic and cook, stirring until fragrant and sizzling but not brown, about 30 seconds. Transfer the garlic and oil to a large bowl. Heat the remaining 2 tablespoons oil in the pan over medium heat. Whisk lemon juice, pepper, and salt into the garlic oil. Add the pasta to the bowl along with sardines, parsley, and parmesan. Gently stir to combine. Serve sprinkled with the parmesan cheese.

Stuffed Roasted Baked Tomatoes with Lentils and Tuna

4 large organic tomato washed, cut in half, and
    scoop the insides out to discard
2 garlic cloves, minced
1 cup green or brown lentils, washed and picked over
1 bay leaf
1/2 medium onion
Salt to taste
1 can water-packed tuna, drained
1/4 cup chopped flat-leaf parsley
1 tablespoon chopped chives
1 tablespoon fresh lemon juice
1 tablespoon sherry vinegar or red wine vinegar
1 teaspoon Dijon mustard
1/4 cup extra-virgin olive oil

Place the lentils, half the garlic, the bay leaf, and the onion in a medium-size dutch oven pot. Add 1 quart water. Bring to a boil; reduce the heat and add salt to taste. Cover and simmer 30 minutes until the lentils are just tender. Remove the onion and bay leaf and discard. Drain the lentils through a strainer set over a bowl. You want to save some broth this way from the lentils.

Meanwhile, wash your tomatoes; cut them in half and scoop out the insides to discard. Set aside. In a large bowl, mix the tuna, parsley, chives, and drained lentils.

In a small bowl, whisk together the lemon juice, vinegar, mustard, remaining garlic clove, and salt and pepper to taste. Whisk in the olive oil and 2 tablespoons of the broth from the lentils. Toss with the tuna and lentils; stuff the tomatoes with the mixture.

Place in an oven-safe glass baking dish. Bake at 350° F for 25 minutes.

Good Ole Salmon Glaze Recipe for the Grill or Oven

Place all the ingredients in a Ziploc bag. Add your salmon and let it marinate overnight or at least 3 hours.

3/4 cup balsamic vinegar
2 tablespoons maple syrup
1 tablespoon Dijon mustard
1 clove garlic, minced
Add peeled minced ginger to taste.

You only need to marinate for a few hours.

SIXTEEN
GLUTEN-FREE
ALCOHOLIC
DRINKS

This by far is my favorite chapter in my book!

Many companies have started to come out with wonderfully delicious gluten-free beers, wines, and all your liquors are gluten-free too!

Coconut-Water Vodka Cocktail

Ice
1 1/2 oz. vodka
6 oz. coconut water

Add a slice of orange, lime, or lemon for garnish and extra flavor

Combine all the wet ingredients in a shaker and shake well for 30 seconds. Pour over ice and add your garnish.

Pink-a-Colada

3 cups cranberry juice cocktail
2 cups coconut water
1 1/2 cups pineapple juice
2 cups coconut rum garnish with a pineapple wedges

Combine all the wet ingredients in a shaker and shake well for 30 seconds. Pour over ice and add your garnish.

Coconut Creamsicle Margaritas

2 oz. Grand Marnier
2 oz. orange juice
1 1/2 oz. tequila (silver)
1 oz. lime juice
1 oz. coconut water
1 oz. light coconut milk (canned)
1 oz. simple syrup or coconut nectar
Toasted coconut
A slice of orange and lime for garnish

To rim glasses, fill a plate with coconut. Rub honey on the rim of glass; turn glasses upside down and coat rim with the coconut. Fill glass with ice.

Combine all the wet ingredients in a shaker and shake well for 30 seconds. Pour over ice and add your garnish.

Pineapple-Coconut Sour

Ice
4 oz. pineapple juice
2 oz. vodka (use a coconut-flavored brand)
1 oz. lime juice
1 fresh lime

Add a few ice cubes in a shaker with a lid. Add the pineapple juice, vodka, and lime juice. Shake for a few moments until it's well chilled and then pour over fresh ice cubes. Garnish with a wedge of lime.

Pumpkin Martin

1 tablespoon pumpkin purée
1 tablespoon coconut milk
1/2 oz. Cointreau

1 1/2 oz. tequila (coconut; regular tequila is fine)
Ice (fresh)
Cinnamon sticks (optional)
Cinnamon (sprinkle)
Red pepper (sprinkle)

Put pumpkin puree, milk, Cointreau, tequila, and ice in a martini shaker and shake until chilled and well blended. Pour into a martini glass. Add cinnamon stick and extra flavor. Sprinkle a dash cinnamon and red pepper for an extra kick on top.

Gin Rickey

2 ounces gin
Juice of 1 lime
Club soda
Lime wedge for garnish

Fill a glass with ice. Pour the gin and lime juice over the ice. Top with club soda. Garnish with a lime wedge.

Combine all the wet ingredients in a shaker and shake well for 30 seconds. Pour over ice and add your garnish

Whiskey Sour

1 1/2 ounces whiskey (or bourbon, Scotch, Canadian whiskey, or Irish whiskey)
4 ounces sour mix (recipe follows)
Crushed ice
1 maraschino cherry

Combine the whiskey and sour mix in a large old-fashioned glass with ice. Stir, garnish with cherry, and serve.

Sour Mix

1 ounce lemon juice
1 ounce sugar

2 ounces water

(Or you can mix the lemon juice with 3 ounces of coconut nectar)

Combine lemon juice and sugar then dilute with water and stir to dissolve sugar.

Mimosa Cocktail

For 1

1/3 cup (79 ml) chilled dry sparkling wine

1/3 cup (79 ml) chilled orange juice (freshly squeezed is best)

1 tablespoon (15 ml) Grand Marnier or triple sec (optional)

Fill 8 champagne flutes 1/2 full with chilled sparkling wine. Top with orange juice. If you are using, top mimosa with 1 tablespoon of Grand Marnier or triple sec.

Cranberry Cosmopolitan

Ice

1 1/2 ounces vodka, preferably ruby-red vodka or citron vodka

1/2 ounce orange liqueur, such as Cointreau or Grand Marnier

3/4 ounce fresh lime juice

1 ounce cranberry juice, red or white (make sure it's high-fructose corn syrup free)

1 fresh or frozen cranberry

To make the cranberry cosmopolitan, fill a cocktail shaker with ice. Measure in the vodka, orange liqueur, and lime and cranberry juices and shake vigorously.

Strain the cranberry cosmopolitan into a martini glass and float a cranberry in the drink for garnish. Repeat as needed.

Classic Bloody Mary

1/4 cup (2 ounces) tomato juice

3 tablespoons (1 1/2 ounces) vodka

1 teaspoon Worcestershire sauce

3/4 teaspoon freshly grated horseradish

3 dashes hot pepper sauce, such as Tabasco
1 pinch salt
1 dash freshly ground black pepper
About 1 cup ice cubes
1/4 teaspoon fresh lemon juice
1 stalk celery
1 lemon wedge (optional)

In a pitcher, stir together tomato juice, vodka, Worcestershire sauce, horseradish, hot sauce, salt, and pepper. Stir well. Fill your glass with ice then pour mixture over the ice into the glass. Sprinkle lemon juice over. Garnish with celery stalk and lemon wedge (if using) and serve.

Chocolate Eruption Cocktail

Chocolate syrup, as needed
1 ounce vodka (use potato vodka for gluten-free)
1 ounce coffee liqueur
1/2 ounce vanilla-almond creamer
2 ounces chocolate-coconut beverage

Drizzle the sides of an empty serving glass with chocolate syrup. Pour remaining ingredients into a cocktail shaker or liquid measuring cup and stir. Pour the mixture into the serving glass and enjoy! Optional: garnish with cocoa power or chocolate sprinkles.

Almond-tini

4 oz. vanilla almond milk and 1/2 oz. vanilla vodka shaken over ice, strained, and poured into a glass swirled with 1 teaspoon chocolate syrup and garnished with a vanilla bean

Vodka Mojito

Fresh mint leaves
Crushed ice
1 teaspoon agave nectar
Squeeze of lime

1 ounce Cîroc vodka
Club soda

Lightly press the fresh mint leaves in a cocktail glass with a muddler. Fill the glass with crushed ice and add the agave nectar, fresh-squeezed lime juice, and vodka; shake. Top off with club soda and garnish with a sprig of mint.

Pink Tequila Cocktails

Freshly squeezed 2 pink grapefruits
2 ounces tequila
1/2 juice from 1 lime

Combine all the ingredients in a shaker and shake well for 30 seconds. Pour over ice and add your garnish.

Oddtini

2 ounces of gin or vodka
3 ounces freshly squeezed pink grapefruit juice
2 ounces club soda
Lime wedge

Combine all the ingredients in a shaker and shake well for 30 seconds. Pour over ice and add your garnish.

Soco Lime

2 ounces southern comfort
2 ounces of freshly squeezed lime juice
3 ounces club soda
Lime wedge

Combine all the ingredients in a shaker and shake well for 30 seconds. Pour over ice and add your garnish.

NONTOXIC HOUSE HOLD CLEANING IDEAS, NATURAL BUG REPELLANT SPRAY, AND A FEW OTHER THINGS.

**** Readers are urged to all appropriate precautions before taking on any *do-it-yourself* task. Always follow the directions and use precautions when making your own homemade products. Never stretch your abilities too far. Each individual, fabric, or material may react differently to particular suggested use. Although this is a nontoxic and natural way to clean your home, always wear protective gloves and eyewear. Although every effort has been made to provide you with the best possible information, neither the publisher nor author are responsible for accidents, injuries, damage incurred as a result of tasks performed by readers. The author will not assume responsibility for personal or property damages from resulting in the use of formulas found in this book. This book is not a substitute for professional services. ****

This homemade laundry detergent recipe not only keeps those harsh chemicals away, but it's also cheaper, lasts longer, and made with all-natural ingredients; it's a greener, healthier alternative to commercial chemically loaded products. There's nothing more natural or better than natural products like vinegar, baking soda, and essential oils.

Homemade Powder Laundry Soap

I mix mine in a large bucket then pour it in a large glass container with a 1/4 small scoop. Only 3 ingredients to make this detergent!

Add 3 cups each of the washing soda and borax detergent booster. Mix well. Grate one bar of FELS-NAPTHA soap in a bowl. (Any castile soap or ivory soap will work too.)

All you need is 1/4 of a cup for each load, and this is exactly the scoop size that I use. Makes things easier for me. Your laundry will be fresh, clean, and actually smell good.

Homemade Liquid Laundry Detergent

 2 gallons + 1 quart boiling water
 1 bar FELS-NAPTHA soap (castile or Ivory soap), grated
 2 cups borax detergent booster
 2 cups Washing Soda
 3-gallon bucket
 Gallon bucket
 Wooden mixing spoon
 Cheese grater

Bring 1 gallon of water to a boil and pour that water into your bucket. Next, add the borax and washing soda and stir to dissolve it completely in the hot water with a wooden spoon.

On your stove, bring 1 quart of water to a boil and add the grated soap to it. You want to melt this completely, so keep stirring until the soap is completely dissolved without any chunks.

Pour the melted soap into your bucket with the already-dissolved borax/washing soda mixture. Stir very well.

Add the last gallon of boiling water to the bucket and stir to mix. The detergent will need to cool down overnight. Use 1/2 cup per load.

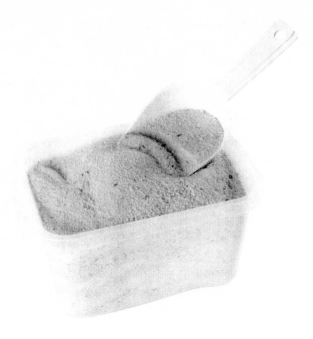

Homemade Dryer Sheets

2 cup of vinegar
20 drops of your favorite essential oil scents
Cut 10 pieces of fabric in wash cloths size squares.
1 glass container with a lid

Mix the vinegar and the essential oil scents in the glass container. Fold your fabric and place in your jar. Give your jar a good shake and mix the solution all over your fabric. After you've already dried your clothes, turn your dryer on the no-heat cycle and put a few of your dryer sheets in your dried load for about 10 minutes. Squeeze out excess liquid. Your dryer sheets should be damp. Don't be afraid to mix essential oils. Lavender, eucalyptus, lemon and rosemary are very refreshing scents when combined.

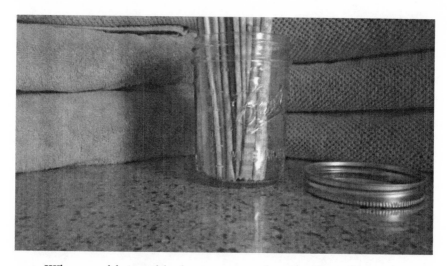

What could possibly be wrong with using store-bought dryer sheets? Let's not forget about all the artificial fragrances. You can do a quick online search on why not to use dryer sheets, and you will end up with a long list of reasons with some pretty interesting chemicals—benzyl acetate, ethyl acetate, chloroform, A-Terpineol, among the others that are neurotoxins, carcinogens, and even listed on the EPA's Hazardous Waste List! For a complete list of what's really in your dryer sheets, along with all their health risks, take a moment with your computer or phone and check out this link: http://www.naturalnews.com/022902.html

Reasons to Ditch Toxic Dryer Sheets

Who doesn't want fantastically smelling clothes? They are awesomely feeling on our skin too. What do you use to accomplish this softening effect? Most likely dryer sheets, right? Or some sort of fabric softener with a wonderful scent.

The Bad News about Dryer Sheets

We use fabric softeners and dryer sheets on a regular, almost-daily, routine. This is a daily routine that, unknowingly, one of the most toxic things we can do. These little fantastic, awesomely smelling sheets are full of toxic chemicals. We put these chemicals all over our clothes. It makes us feel great, by smelling great, which in turn get on all over skin—and most importantly, get absorbed "into our body" from our skin. This "into our body" absorption contributes to poisoning our nervous system. These toxic chemicals will build up in our bodies and over time can wreak havoc on our nervous system.

Have you taken the time to read and research the ingredients in dryer sheets?

According to the author of *The Brain Wash*, here are the seven most common chemicals found in dryer sheets and their effect on the central nervous system:

1. Alpha-Terpineol causes central nervous system disorders. Can also cause loss of muscular coordination, central nervous system depression, and headache.

2. Benzyl alcohol causes central nervous system disorders, headaches, nausea, vomiting, dizziness, central nervous system depression, and, in severe cases, death.

3. Camphor is on the US EPA's Hazardous Waste list. Central nervous system stimulant that causes dizziness, confusion, nausea, twitching muscles, and convulsions.

4. Chloroform is on the EPA's Hazardous Waste list. Neurotoxic and carcinogenic.

5. Ethyl Acetate is on the EPA's Hazardous Waste list. Narcotic. May cause headaches and narcosis (stupor).

6. Linalool causes central nervous system disorders. Narcotic. In studies of animals, it caused ataxic gait (loss of muscular coordination), reduced spontaneous motor activity, and depression.

7. Pentane causes headaches, nausea, vomiting, dizziness, drowsiness, and loss of consciousness. Repeated inhalation of vapors causes central nervous system depression.

After reading this, will this be enough information to make you think twice about those store-bought dryer sheets and fabric softeners?

Homemade Deodorant

I've been making my own deodorant for years. It all started when I came across an article on the Internet about how aluminum-based antiperspirants may increase the risk for breast cancer, Alzheimer's disease and kidney disease. (Scientists noticed that dialysis patients who had these high aluminum levels were more likely to develop dementia too.) Our bodies are supposed to sweat. Sweat isn't inherently stinky either. In fact, it's nearly odorless. The stench comes from bacteria that break down from one of two types of sweat on your skin. Deodorant advertisers have done a pretty neat job of convincing us that we're disgustingly smelly people who in fact need to be refined and save our stinky selves by their products. We've been wonderfully brainwashed into thinking sweating is a bad thing. Sweating from the heat, sweating from exercise, and sweating from stress are all different, chemically speaking. Stress sweat smells the worst. That's because smelly sweat is only produced by one of the two types of sweat glands called the apocrine glands, which are usually in areas with lots of hair—like our armpits, the groin area, and scalp. The odor is the result of the bacteria that break down the sweat once it's released onto your skin. Fun fact: While women have more sweat glands than men, men's sweat glands produce more sweat.

1/2 cup baking soda
1/2 cup arrowroot powder or 1/2 cup of cornstarch
5 tablespoon unrefined virgin coconut oil
10 drops of grapefruit essential oil or lavender essential oil
(You can pick your favorite scent. I like lavender or grapefruit.)

Mix baking soda and arrowroot together. Melt your coconut oil in the microwave in a microwave-safe bowl. Mix all ingredients (the baking soda and arrowroot powder) with the oil. Pour into clean small mason jar. Add your essential oil to the mason jar; close with the lid. Give it a good shake to combine the essential oil with the other mixture. By doing it this way, you can still use that bowl to eat with. Once you mix that essential oil in the bowl, it can only be used for the purpose of making your deodorant. Everything you've used is edible except the essential oils.

This will take roughly 24 hours to set. It will thicken up. I use my finger to scrape what I need and scoop it across my underarm.

Vinegar of the Four-Thieves Insect Repellent

Some of you might not have ever heard of the legend of the Four Thieves Vinegar. This was a time when the bubonic plague was wreaking havoc in Europe. A garlic-vinegar preparation known as the four thieves was credited with protecting many of the people when a plague struck Marseilles, France in 1722. Some say that the preparation originated with four thieves who confessed that they used it with complete protection against the plague while they robbed the bodies of the dead. This mixture is very strong and has antiviral and antibacterial properties. This vinegar makes an effective natural disinfectant spray for household cleaning and also a great bug spray.

> 1 16 ounces of Bragg's Organic Apple Cider Vinegar
> 1 tablespoon each of dried sage, rosemary, lavender,
>   thyme, and mint
> At least quart-size glass jar with airtight lid

Put the vinegar and dried herbs into large mason jar. Seal tightly and store on counter where you can see it each day. Make sure you shake it each day for the next 4 weeks. Remember, vinegar is strong enough to corrode some metal lids, so to avoid this from happening, put plastic wrap on top and then put the lid on or just use a plastic lid.

After 4 weeks, strain the herbs out and store in marked spray bottles and keep it in the fridge until needed. When you use it on your skin, dilute half with water in a spray bottle.

All-Natural Homemade Scouring Powder

> 1 cup baking soda
> 1/2 cup sea salt (commercially made table
>   salt is good for something!)
> 1/2 cup borax detergent booster powder

Pour ingredients into a large mason jar. Seal the lid tightly and shake well to combine.

You can make scouring powder mix a neat little shaker by safely poking some holes in the top with a sharp serrated knife. Or take the lid, place it on a sturdy wood surface (where you don't mind dent and dings), take a screwdriver and a hammer, and hammer several holes in the lid.

Wet the area with undiluted white vinegar. Sprinkle powder on and let sit 10 minutes. Scrub the area with a good scrubbing brush until clean and rinse with vinegar. Mark you jar with a permanent marker: Scouring Powder.

Homemade Oven Cleaner Recipe

1 tablespoon borax detergent booster
1/2 cup vinegar
1/8 cup Dr. Bonner's Castile soap
1 cup boiling water

Combine everything in a spray bottle. Mix well. Sprinkle the inside of your oven with baking soda. Spray a thick layer of the oven cleaner all around your oven. Sprinkle more with baking soda on top of that. Leave overnight. Using a hot wet sponge with a scrubber on one side of, it scrub out in the morning and then proceed to wipe out with a hot, wet rag.

How to Unclog a Drain with Baking Soda and Vinegar

Pour a large pot of boiling-hot water down your drain. Pour 1/2 cup baking soda in the drain as best as you can. Let that sit for a few minutes. Next, pour a mixture of 1 cup vinegar and then 1 cup of very hot water down on top of the baking soda. Allow it to sit for 5–10 minutes. Pour one last time with boiling water, and the drain should be clear.

Homemade Glass Cleaner

1/4 cup rubbing alcohol

1/4 cup white vinegar
1 tablespoon cornstarch
2 cups warm water

Combine everything in a spray bottle and shake well. Shake well before using too, as the cornstarch would have settled at the bottom (and subsequently plug the spray mechanism if it's not mixed in well).

Natural Disinfectant

This natural disinfectant can clean germs that cause food-borne illness on your kitchen countertops. Tea tree oil is a naturally occurring essential oil with antifungal properties that can kill staphylococcus, E-coli, and salmonella. The vinegar has acid qualities that also help to kill germs and reduce microbial growth. The castile soap gives it an extra cleansing boost.

2 cups of water
20 drops of tea tree oil
1 cup white distilled vinegar
1 teaspoon Dr. Bonner's liquid castile soap

Fill your bottle with water; pour in your tea tree oil and add the vinegar. Mix well. Next, add your castile soap. Put the sprayer on the bottle; seal tightly and shake. You can label your bottle with a black magic marker: Kitchen Cleaner.

Shower Glass Soap Scum Remover and a Bathroom Disinfectant

Borax is a naturally occurring powder consisting of sodium, boron, and oxygen. It's a very powerful disinfectant. It also will not harm septic systems or plumbing.

3 cups of warm water in a spray bottle
2 tablespoons of borax detergent booster
5 tablespoons of distilled vinegar
1/2 teaspoon of Dr. Bonner's liquid castile soap
10 drops of tea tree oil

Fill your bottle with the very warm water. Pour your borax detergent booster in and shake to dissolve. Next, add your vinegar and liquid castile soap. Mix well. Spray on your glass or the area you want to disinfect. Leave for 10–30 minutes. For hard soap scum, you will have to take a scrub brush and scrub over that area and rinse with water. If you're using it as a disinfectant, spray area and leave on for 30 minutes then wipe off with a wet nonmicrobial cloth. Don't forget to label your spray bottle with a black permanent marker.

The Tipsy Lavender-and-Lemon Bathroom Disinfecting Spray

1/2 cup white vinegar
1/2 cup vodka
10 drops lavender essential oil
10 drops lemon essential oil
1 1/2 cups water

Fill your bottle with water; add your drops of lavender and lemon essential oils. Next, add your vodka and white vinegar. Mix well. Spray on your bathroom surfaces and let sit for 10–30 minutes. Wipe off with a nonmicrobial cloth. Don't forget to label your spray bottle with a black permanent marker.

Bathroom Mold Disinfecting Spray

You don't have to grab bleach to get rid of mold in your bathroom. This 3 combo all-natural mixture will do the trick. I would spray the areas in my bathroom and leave it on for 10 minutes and wipe the moldy areas away. Vodka might be a little bit pricey, but you won't be breathing in toxic chemicals or having to worry about your skin absorbing a list of toxic chemicals. Vinegar is naturally antimicrobial; tea tree is natural fungicide, which can eliminate any mold or mildew problems and kills black mold spores! Don't forget to label your spray bottle with a black permanent marker.

1 cup of white vinegar
1 cup of vodka
20 drops of tea tree oil

No diluting this combo. Mix well in a spray bottle and label with Bathroom Mold Killer. Spray onto hard surfaces where mold and mildew are growing and let this amazing combo go to work. You'll still have to scrub a bit, but with repeated use, this all-natural cleaner will kill the fungus and help to prevent future growth. Shake each time before use.

Natural Wood Floor Cleaner

> 1/2 cup distilled white vinegar
> 1/2 cup of EVOO
> Juice from 1 lemon

Mix well and rub lightly onto floors to bring back shine and clean spots. Add a few drops of essential oil of choice for nice scent. Make sure to wipe off completely to avoid slippery floors!

Natural All-Purpose Floor Cleaner

> 2 cup distilled vinegar
> 2 cups water
> 4 cups of water
> 4 tablespoons of washing soda

Mix the washing soda with 4 cups of water in a bucket. Dampen you mop with the mixture. Mop well. Next, rinse mop with regular water. Pour out mixture, rinse bucket, and place regular water in the bucket and go over the mopped area. Next, place the 2 cups of vinegar and 2 cups of water mixture in a bucket and dampen the mop. Mop well.

Spotless Floor Cleaner

> 1 cup of white vinegar
> 1 tablespoon of liquid dish soap
> 1 cup of baking soda
> 2 gallons of very warm tap water

Pour the very warm tap water in your bucket. Add your baking soda, dish soap, and white vinegar. Mop well. Next, rinse mop with regular water. Pour out mixture, rinse bucket, and place regular water in the bucket and go over the mopped area. It will leave your floor smelling amazing and clean.

Nontoxic Homemade Beeswax Candles

Nothing like a clean house with a great-smelling scented candle burning. Beeswax emits negative ions, which helps to cleanse the air. Most commercial candles are made from paraffin wax, and when heated, this wax releases two nasty chemicals that are also found in diesel fuel: benzene and toluene. These two are found in the sooty residue of burning candles. Benzene is cancer causing and toluene affects the central nervous system. The wicks that most scented candles have contain lead, and when lit, a lead wick emits five times the amount of lead categorized as dangerous for children (a level set by the EPA). Exposure to lead is associated with learning and behavior problems and a hormone disruption. Lead wicks were banned in 2003, but some candle companies still use them.

Oh, and that delightful smell that comes from commercial candles is due to artificial fragrances? There are 3,163 ingredients that hide behind the word *fragrance*. Here is an alternative way to help cleanse the air and do it a nontoxic way. If you don't want to make your own beeswax candles, there are plenty of companies who sell them. Go to my blog website http://thehypothyroidismchick.com/ and check out my blog on beeswax candles.

Nontoxic Homemade Beeswax Candles

1/2 pound organic beeswax
1/2 cup raw coconut oil
Cotton wicks (size medium)
25 drops of your favorite essential oil scent
Mason jars (this will make 2 8-ounce candles)

In a double boiler, melt the beeswax and the coconut oil together. You can prepare your jars with the wick by wrapping the top end of the wick around a pencil, or place two chopsticks around the wick to hold it in place.

The goal is to get the wick to stay in the middle of the jar as we pour in the beeswax and it sets. It doesn't matter the method as long as the wick stays in the center of the jar. Once the wax and oil are melted, fill each jar carefully and slowly so the wick stays in place. Allow the wax to set for 2 days before lighting.

Indoor air quality is essential to help with our overall health and well-being. It's not enough to be aware of all the outdoor chemicals that we are exposed to every day, but inside our home, we can have more control. We are a walking human chemical experiment for companies, and they don't care about our health, just lining their pockets with money. A little common sense can go a long way. We can be more aware about using chemical cleaners, paints, glues and pesticides, and use products that don't pollute. Look for a greener products. Research, research, and research. I can't stress this enough. Call and ask the companies about their products. Household cleaners, dust, paints, bug sprays, smoke from cooking or cigarettes, and fibers from some building materials all can make indoor air unhealthy to breathe. We can take a stand for our health. Stop using commercial products that are laced with unknown and harmful, body-damaging products. Use better ventilation filters, salt lamps, bamboo charcoal bags, and have indoor plants that naturally purify the air. Open a window! Let some fresh air in. Having good indoor air quality is very important, especially since many of us spend so much time inside. NASA did a study to find out which plants were best to filter the air of the space station. They had several listed, but here are eight. These plants were beneficial to reducing indoor air pollutions and they are as follows: spider plants, philodendron, bamboo palm, snake plant, peace lily, English ivy, golden pothos, and the aloe plant.

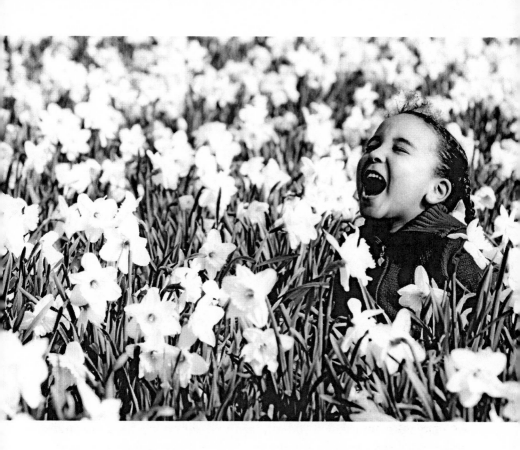

Let's kick hypothyroidisms booty the slow-cooker way! Here are a few recipes **from my next book**. Look for it in stores or order it online in the near future. No time to be in the kitchen? Do you need foods that promote thyroid health? Heal your body from the inside out with over one hundred and one (101) hypothyroidism-nourishing recipes that cook themselves.

A Survivor's Cookbook:
Guide to Kicking Hypothyroidism's Booty
the Slow Cooker Way.

Overnight Slow Cooker Apple-Cinnamon Oatmeal

    4 cups water
    1 1/2 cups apple juice
    2 cup steel-cut oats

1 teaspoon ground cinnamon
1/2 teaspoon grated fresh ginger or 1/4 teaspoon ground ginger
1/4 teaspoon salt
2 medium apples, coarsely chopped
Honey

Cover and cook on low heat, setting for 6 to 7 hours.

Slow Cooker Mexican Rice with Black Beans

1 cup of brown rice
2 cups vegetable broth
1/2 cup cilantro
2 cloves Garlic
1 4-ounce) can green chiles
1 (14.5 ounce) can Petite diced tomatoes
1 can black beans, rinsed and drained
1 sweet onion, chopped
1 teaspoon cumin
1 tablespoon of EVOO

In a large cast-iron skillet, add oil; turn to medium-low heat and sauté onion until tender, about 4 minutes. Add garlic and continue to sauté 1 additional minute. Add remaining ingredients and transfer to a crock pot—2 hours on high, 4 hours on low.

Slow Cooker Taco Soup

1 pound ground turkey
1 15.5-ounce can black-eyed peas
1 15-ounce can organic black beans
1 15-ounce can organic chili beans
1 15-ounce can organic garbanzo beans
1 14.5-ounce can Mexican-style stewed tomatoes
1 11-ounce can whole kernel corn with sweet peppers
1 1.25-ounce package taco seasoning mix, low sodium

Brown ground turkey in a cast-iron skillet. Add cooked ground turkey, undrained vegetables, and taco seasoning mix and mix. Cover and cook on low heat setting for 6 to 8 hours or on high heat setting for 3 to 4 hours.

Slow Cooker Buffalo Chicken Chili

1.5 pounds organic ground chicken
1 large onion
2 medium stalks of celery, diced
2 medium carrots, peeled and diced
1 28-ounce can fire-roasted diced tomatoes
1 15-ounce can white beans, rinsed and drained
2 teaspoon chili powder
2 teaspoon cumin
1 cup chicken broth
1/4 cup buffalo wing sauce
1/2 teaspoon salt
1/2 teaspoon pepper

In a cast-iron skillet, sauté onion until soft for about 5 minutes. Add the ground chicken, celery, and carrots and cook until meat begins to brown, about 4–5 minutes. Remove the meat and vegetables from the pan and transfer into the slow cooker. Add tomatoes, beans, spices, salt, and pepper. Pour in chicken broth and hot sauce and stir. Set slow cooker to low, cover, and cook for 5–6 hours.

Slow Cooker Buffalo Chicken Lettuce Wraps

For the chicken:

6 boneless skinless chicken breast
1 celery stalk, diced
1/2 onion, diced
1 tablespoon of nonsoy, nondairy butter
1 clove garlic
1/2 cup of low-sodium chicken broth
1 12-ounce bottle of Frank's wing sauce
1 packet of organic dry ranch dressing mix

For the wraps:

6 large lettuce leaves, Bibb or iceberg

Place chicken breasts in slow cooker. Sprinkle ranch seasoning over chicken then pour in hot sauce and chicken stock. Add the diced onions, celery, and garlic. Make sure your chicken is completely covered in liquid. Turn chicken a few times until it is coated and everything is mixed together.

Cook on low for 5–6 hours. Once cooked, take chicken out and shred in a bowl. After your chicken has been shredded, add in 1 tablespoon of butter to the crock pot and let it melt. Add some of your liquid from the slow cooker to the chicken until you get the flavor you want. This also keeps the chicken moist.

Slow Cooker Two-Bean Chili

    1 large onion (chopped)
    2 small green peppers (or 1 medium) chopped
    Olive oil spray
    1 pound extra lean ground turkey
    1 teaspoon garlic powder
    1 teaspoon onion powder
    salt and pepper
    2 15-ounce cans organic pinto beans (drained and rinsed)
    1 15-ounce can organic black beans (drained and rinsed)
    1 28-ounce can diced tomatoes
    1 15-ounce can tomato sauce
    1 tablespoon tomato paste (I like to freeze the leftover paste in a
        small Ziploc freezer bag, divided into tablespoon section,
        and just grab a chunk when needed)
    2 cups water
    2 teaspoon chili powder

Add chopped onions and green peppers to a cast-iron skillet sprayed with olive oil spray and cook until onions are translucent and peppers are soft. Add ground beef, garlic powder, onion powder, salt, and pepper and sauté until turkey is thoroughly cooked.

Add turkey mixture to crock pot and all the remaining ingredients to the slow cooker; mix well.

Cook on high for 4 hours or low for 6–8 hours.

Slow Cooker Butter and Garlic Baked Potatoes

Wash your organic potatoes as you normally would for baked potatoes. Next, slice each potato into 3 sections but not all the way cut through. In each slice of the potato, put a thin slice of butter or garlic. I typically alternate with garlic, butter, garlic.

Place the potatoes in the slow cooker top with sliced onions. Let the potatoes slow cook on high for 4 hours.

Slow Cooker Pinto Beans

1 pound dry pinto beans
6 cups water or vegetable broth
1 onion, diced
1 1/2 teaspoon Celtic sea salt
Black pepper to taste
1 bay leaf

Rinse your beans and sort through them looking for bad beans, small rocks, or debris.

In a pot or bowl, add warm water covering the beans by two inches. Let soak overnight. Drain the next day and add beans to a crockpot. Add 6 cups water or broth, bay leaf, and 1 diced onion. Cook on low for 7–9 hours or on high for 4–5 hours.

After beans are tender, add salt and pepper to taste.

Slow Cooker White Chicken Chili

6 cups low-sodium chicken broth
4 cups cooked shredded chicken
2 15-ounce cans great northern beans, drained and rinsed
2 cups salsa verde
2 teaspoon ground cumin

You can top this with diced avocado, chopped fresh cilantro, shredded goat's cheese, chopped green onions, and crumbled gluten-free tortilla chips.

Add everything to the slow cooker and stir to combine. Cook on low for 6–8 hours, or high for 3–4 hours.

Slow Cooker White Bean Soup

2 tablespoons olive oil
4 cloves garlic, minced
1 medium yellow onion, diced
1/2 pound carrots, diced
4 stalks celery, diced
1 pound dry navy beans, rinsed
1 whole bay leaf
1 teaspoon dried rosemary
1/2 teaspoon dried thyme
1/2 teaspoon smoked paprika
Freshly cracked pepper (15–20 cranks of a mill)
1 1/2 teaspoon Himalayan salt
2 32-ounce of low-sodium vegetable broth

Sort through the beans and remove any debris or stones. Give them a quick rinse and then add them to the slow cooker, along with everything else that has been prepped, and add the bay leaf, rosemary, thyme, paprika, and some freshly cracked pepper.

Slow Cooker Garlic Artichokes

4 medium artichokes
4 tablespoons minced fresh garlic, divided
4 tablespoons balsamic vinegar, divided
1/2 cup dry white wine or chicken broth
4 teaspoons extra-virgin olive oil, divided

Cut 1/2 inch off the top of each artichoke and rinse the artichoke. Trim the stem end so the artichoke will stand flat. Pull the leaves back to make it open more to hold the filling.

Place 1 tablespoon of the garlic evenly between the leaves of each artichoke. Place artichokes in slow cooker. Drizzle each artichoke with 1 tablespoon of the vinegar. Pour wine into the slow cooker and add enough water to come up to one-fourth the sides of the artichokes and season with freshly grown pepper. Cook on high 4 hours until the leaves peel off easily away from the base.

Slow Cooker Artichoke Chicken

4 large chicken breasts
1/2 stick of nondairy, nonsoy butter
3 teaspoon minced garlic
1 cup chicken broth
8 ounces fresh mushrooms, sliced
1 14-ounce can artichoke hearts, chopped into quarters
1 teaspoon crushed red pepper
1 teaspoon parsley
Sea salt to taste
Black pepper to taste

Place the chicken in the bottom of the slow cooker. Season with a little sea salt and pepper.

Add artichokes and mushrooms on top of the chicken. Next add the broth, garlic, and spices. Cook on low for 6 hours.

Slow Cooker Butternut Squash Soup

1 medium butternut squash (1 lb of peeled and cubed butternut squash)
1 medium onion, diced
1/2 pound carrots, peeled and cut into chunks
1 Granny Smith apple, peeled and sliced
3 cups vegetable broth
1 bay leaf
1 teaspoon salt
1 teaspoon pepper
1/4 teaspoon dried ground sage
1 13.5-ounce can coconut milk

Salt and pepper to taste

Combine squash, onion, carrots, apple, broth and bay leaf in slow cooker. Cover and cook on low for about 6 hours or until veggies are soft.

Remove bay leaf and discard. Transfer contents of slow cooker to a blender and blend until smooth (or you can use an immersion blender).

When smooth, pour contents back into the slow cooker and add in salt, pepper, sage, and coconut milk. Stir. Taste and then add more salt and pepper to taste.

Slow Cooker Black Bean and Butternut Squash Chili

1 tablespoon plus 2 teaspoons extra-virgin olive oil
1 medium to large butternut squash, peeled and diced
1 large onion, diced
4 cloves garlic, minced
2 tablespoons chili powder
4 teaspoons ground cumin
1/2 teaspoon ground chipotle chili
1/4 teaspoon salt
2 1/2 cups water
2 15-ounce cans black beans, rinsed
1 14-ounce can diced tomatoes
4 teaspoons lime juice
1/2 cup chopped fresh cilantro

Place all ingredients in a slow cooker. Stir well to combine. Cover and cook on high for 4 hours or low for 6 hours.

Squash, Chickpea, and Red Lentil Stew

2 cans of chickpeas, drained and rinsed
2 1/2 butternut squash, peeled, seeded,
    and cut into 1-inch cubes
2 large carrots, peeled and cut into bite-size pieces
1 large onion, chopped
1 cup red lentils

4 cups vegetable broth
2 tablespoons tomato paste
1 tablespoon minced, peeled fresh ginger
1 1/2 teaspoons ground cumin
1 teaspoon salt
1/4 teaspoon freshly ground pepper
1/4 cup lime juice
1/4 cup packed fresh cilantro leaves, chopped

Combine the soaked chickpeas, squash, carrots, onion, lentils, broth, tomato paste, ginger, cumin, salt, and pepper in a 6-quart slow cooker. Put on the lid and cook on low until the chickpeas are tender and the lentils have begun to break down, 5 to 6 1/2 hours.

Slow Cooker Brown Lentil Chili

1 medium onion, diced
3 cloves garlic, minced
1 jalapeño, diced, seeds removed
1 red pepper, chopped
1 yellow pepper, chopped
1 large carrot, peeled and diced
2 1/2 cups vegetable broth
2 15-ounce cans tomato sauce
2 15-ounce cans diced tomatoes
1 16-ounce bag brown lentils, rinsed
2 15-ounce cans small red beans, rinsed and drained
2–3 tablespoons chili powder (we used 3 tablespoons)
1 tablespoon cumin
Celtic sea salt or Himalayan sea salt and black pepper, to taste

Place all ingredients in a slow cooker. Stir well to combine. Cover and cook on high for 4 hours or low for 6 hours.

Slow Cooker Yellow Lentil Dahl

2 cups dried yellow lentils, rinsed and sorted

1 tablespoon olive oil
1 onion, diced
4 garlic cloves, minced
2 tablespoons fresh ginger, finely chopped
1 tablespoon garam masala
1 tablespoon curry powder
1 teaspoon ground cumin
1 teaspoon ground coriander
1 teaspoon mustard powder
1 teaspoon ground turmeric
4 cups vegetable broth
1 14.5-ounce can crushed tomatoes

Rinse the lentils in cold running water. Sift through and remove any small stones or debris. Heat the olive oil in a cast-iron skillet over medium heat. Add the onion, garlic, and fresh ginger and sauté until the onion is softened, about 5 minutes.

Add the sautéed onion mixture, lentils, all the spices, vegetable stock, and tomatoes into the slow cooker. Cook on high for about 4 hours or low for 6 hours.

Slow Cooker Red Lentil Soup

1 tablespoon olive oil
1 large white or yellow onion, chopped
2 carrots, peeled and chopped
2 celery stalks, chopped
4 cloves garlic, minced
2 teaspoons ground cumin
1/2 teaspoon cayenne pepper
1 1/2 teaspoons smoked paprika
4 cups dry red lentils, picked over for debris and rinsed
2 bay leaves
2 32-ounce containers of low-sodium vegetable stock
Celtic sea salt or Himalayan sea salt

This tastes great with a splash of red wine vinegar, with sprinkled some minced raw red onion and some minced fresh cilantro leaves.

Heat olive oil in a cast-iron skillet over medium heat. Sauté onions, carrots, and celery and cook, stirring frequently about 5 minutes. Add garlic and cook an additional 1 minute. Then stir in cumin, cayenne, and paprika and continue cooking until fragrant.

Transfer mixture to a slow cooker. Add lentils, bay leaves, and the stock. Stir in to season 1 teaspoon of salt and cover. Set slow cooker to low and cook for 4 hours, stirring once each hour and adding in additional broth as needed to maintain a loose, soup-like consistency.

Use an immersion blender or transfer in batches to a blender. Purée until smooth. Ladle into bowls and top with red onion, splash of red vinegar and cilantro.

Slow Cooker Southwestern Pinto Bean Soup

  2 cups dry pinto beans
  5 cups cold water
  2 14-ounce cans reduced-sodium vegetable broth
  1/2 cup water
  1 large onion, chopped
  3 cloves garlic, minced
  2 tablespoons of Mrs. Dash southwestern chipotle seasoning
      blend (this makes it a little bit spicy; if 2 tablespoons is too
      much, just adjust to your taste)
  1 teaspoon ground cumin
  1/4 teaspoon cayenne pepper
  1 14.5-ounce can fire-roasted diced tomatoes, undrained
  Snipped fresh cilantro and/or sliced green onions (optional)

Cover and cook on low-heat setting for 8 to 10 hours or on high-heat setting for 4 to 5 hours. Stir in undrained tomatoes; cover and cook for 30 minutes more.

If desired, partially mash mixture with a potato masher, leaving soup chunky.

Slow Cooker Spaghetti Squash and Turkey Meatballs

Spaghetti squash is an excellent, low-carb alternative to pasta.

1 medium spaghetti squash.
1 pound of ground organic turkey.
1 can of tomato sauce (I used a 14 ounce can)
2 tablespoons of hot pepper relish
4 to 6 cloves of garlic, minced
2 tablespoons of olive oil.
2 teaspoons of Italian seasoning

Put your tomato sauce, olive oil, garlic, hot pepper relish, and Italian seasoning into your slow cooker and give it a good stir. Wash your squash then proceed to cut your squash in half and scoop out the seeds. Place your 2 squash halves face down into your slow cooker.

In a bowl add ground turkey, 2 tablespoons of minced garlic, 1 tablespoon of Italian seasoning. Roll your ground turkey into meatballs then fit as many as you can in the sauce around the squash. Make sure you get them in the sauce covered. Cook on high for 4 hours or cook on low for 6 hours.

After 4–6 hours, carefully pull your squash out; it will be hot and very soft. I use two forks, one to stick in each side. Once placed on a plate or bowl, use a large fork to pull the "spaghetti" out of your squash, place in a bowl, then top with your meatballs and sauce.

Slow Cooker Navy Bean

Navy beans are a very good source of folate, manganese, protein, vitamin B1, phosphorus, copper, magnesium iron and high in fiber. Navy beans are naturally high in *iodine*. Just 1/2 cup of these beans contain about 32/mcg of iodine.

1 pound bag of dried beans, rinsed and picked over to check for debris such as rocks and sticks
1 onion, diced
2 32-ounce vegetable broth
1 teaspoon of Himalayan sea salt
1 teaspoon of pepper

Cover and cook on low-heat setting for 8 to 10 hours or on high-heat setting for 4 to 5 hours. Serve over a bed of brown rice.

Slow Cooker Zesty Lemon Herb Turkey Breast

Turkey is rich in protein, low in fat, and is a source of iron, zinc, potassium, phosphorus, vitamin B6, and niacin. It also contains the amino acid tryptophan, selenium, and is lower on the GI index scale.

> 2 turkey London breast, 2–3 pounds
> Juice and zest of two lemons
> 1 teaspoon of dried rosemary
> 1 teaspoon of dried sage
> 2 tablespoons of Dijon mustard
> 1 whole onion sliced
> Himalayan sea salt and pepper to taste

Place the turkey tenderloin in the bottom of the slow cooker. In a bowl, mix everything but the onions and rub the mixture completely over the turkey breast.

Next, after the mixture is completely covered on the turkey breast. Place the onions rings all over the turkey. Cover and cook for 8 hours on low. After it has been cooked, don't eat the skin. It's very high in fat. We just left it on for the extra flavoring. This would be great with a side of quinoa or brown rice.

Slow Cooker Wild Rice with Cranberries and Mushrooms

Wild rice has a wonderfully gluten-free nutty flavor and is actually considered an edible grass. It has twice as much protein as brown rice, is very rich in antioxidants, has high fiber content, has essential minerals such as phosphorus, zinc, magnesium, and folate, vitamins A, C, and E. Wild rice could even turn out to be one of nature's superfoods. In Chinese medicine, wild rice is used as a treatment for diabetes for it might help to reduce insulin resistance.

White button mushrooms can help enhance weight loss, and it's a good source of vitamin D; it has anti-inflammatory benefits, excellent for diabetics, helps to protect liver and kidneys, increases blood flow, helps normalize cholesterol levels. Mushrooms contain loads of vitamin B2 and vitamin B3 (niacin), just enough to jump start that metabolism.

Dried cranberries has antioxidants and can help reduce inflammation. Sounds like this dish is one of those must-eat for your health! Who knew being healthy can taste so good?

1 1/2 cups uncooked wild rice
1 tablespoon ghee or coconut oil, melted
1/4 teaspoon Celtic sea salt or pink Himalayan sea salt
1/4 teaspoon pepper
1/4 cup red onion, diced
2 cans (14 ounces each) vegetable broth
1/2 cup of white button mushrooms, diced
1/2 cup slivered almonds
1/3 cup dried cranberries

Rinse the wild rice in cold water in a mesh strainer. Sauté the onions in 1 teaspoon of coconut oil or ghee. Mix all ingredients except almonds and cranberries. Cover with lid and allow to cook on low-heat setting for 5 hours until wild rice is tender. In ungreased cast-iron skillet, heat almonds over medium-low heat for 5 to 7 minutes, stirring frequently until they start to brown. Once they begin to brown, keep stirring until golden brown and smelling wonderfully fragrant. Stir in almonds and cranberries into rice mixture. Cover and cook on low heat for additional 15 minutes.

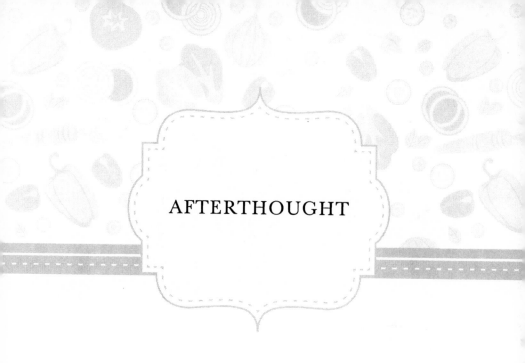

AFTERTHOUGHT

(My final words of encouragement, wisdom, and well-being)

Let's try to simplify our lives. We are so bombarded with consumerism, surrounded by chemicals, and taken aback by this crazy pace of our high-tech, fast-paced digital world. It seems like we've disconnected to get more connected. Try to talk daily *walks* to get fresh air and clear your mind. Plant a garden, start cooking from scratch, clean your house with things that are nontoxic, don't eat anything your great-great-great-grandmother wouldn't recognize as food, keep a journal, reduce your personal stress, and smile more. Be your game-changer. Watch what comes out of your mouth. Don't speak discouragement, sickness, poorness, self-doubt on yourself. Majority of us (thin, fat, tall, short) all battled with something that we don't like about ourselves and want to fix. Enjoy life today; there is no dress rehearsal. Lastly, be you. Nobody does you quite like you do you.

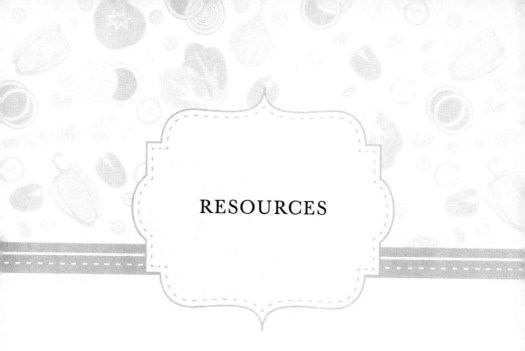

RESOURCES

http://www.healthaliciousness.com/articles/high-tyrosine-foods.php

http://articles.mercola.com/sites/articles/archive/2015/03/21/apple-cider-vinegar-uses.aspx

1 2 12 MedGenMed. 2006; 8(2): 61.

3 6 14 Journal of Food Science May 8, 2014

4 Diabetes Care. 2004 Jan;27(1):281–2.

5 Diabetes Care November 2007 vol. 30 no. 11 2814–2815

7 Bioscience, Biotechnology, and Biochemistry, 65(12) 2690–2694

8 Biosci Biotechnol Biochem. 2001 Dec;65(12):2690–4.

9 J Agric Food Chem. 2011 Jun 22;59(12):6638–44.

10 J Am Diet Assoc. 2005 Dec;105(12):1939–42.

11 Eur J Clin Nutr. 2005 Sep;59(9):983–8.

13 *Reader's Digest*

15 16 Mamavation January 26, 2015

https://www.nlm.nih.gov/medlineplus/druginfo/natural/1002.html#Description

http://cfpub.epa.gov/si/si_public_record_report.cfm?dirEntryId=20899

http://www.ewg.org/enviroblog/2010/02/3163-ingredients-hide-behind-word-fragrance

http://www.lung.org/associations/charters/mid-atlantic/air-quality/indoor-air-quality.html

http://www.washington.edu/news/2008/07/23/toxic-chemicals-found-in-common-scented-laundry-products-air-fresheners/

http://kids.niehs.nih.gov/explore/pollute/dust1_indoor_air.htm

http://www.epa.gov/iaq/pdfs/aircleaners.pdf

https://en.wikipedia.org/wiki/Hygroscopy

Thayer, R. E. (1989). *Biopsychology of Mood and Arousal*. New York: Oxford University Press

Diamond, M. (1988) *Enriching Heredity: The Impact of the Environment on the Anatomy of the Brain*. New York: Free Press.

Yepsen, R. B., Jr. (1987) How to Boost Your Brain Power: Achieving Peak Intelligence, Memory and Creativity. Emmaus, Pa.: Rodale. webmd.com/balance/features/negative-ions-create-positive-vibes

http://wholegrainscouncil.org/whole-grains-101/gluten-free-whole-grains

Wheat Belly—an Analysis of Selected Statements and Basic Theses from the Book"

Julie Jones, Cereal Foods World. July-August 2013, 57(4):177–189.

"Does Wheat Make Us Fat and Sick?"

Fred Brouns et al., Journal of Cereal Science. 58(2013) 209–15.

Rolls BJ, Roe LS, Beach AM, Kris-Etherton PM. Provision of foods differing in energy density affects long-term weight loss. Obesity Research 2005;13:1052–1060.

http://www.secretofthieves.com/four-thieves-vinegar.cfm

Nature's Medicines, Richard Lucas, 1966, p38

Rolls BJ, Roe LS, Meengs JS. Reducing the energy density and portion size of foods decreases energy intake over two days. ObesityResearch 2004;12:A5. 32.

Rolls BJ, Morris EL, Roe LS. Portion size of food affects energy intake in normal-weight and overweight men and women. American Journal of Clinical Nutrition 2002;76:12071213

US Department of Health and Human Services, US Department of Agriculture. Dietary Guidelines for Americans 2005. 6th ed. Washington, D.C., 2005

Early citation of "Forthave's Vinegar" The Mirror of Literature, Amusement, and Instruction, Volume 12, 1828, p89

https://www.organicfacts.net/health-benefits/herbs-and-spices/onion.html

http://www.drfuhrman.com/library/cruciferous_vegetables_and_thyroid.aspx

http://livingtraditionally.com/turmeric-drink-can-revolutionize-health/

http://thecoconutmama.com/2014/01/how-much-coconut-oil-should-you-eat-a-day/

http://authoritynutrition.com/why-are-eggs-good-for-you/

http://slism.com/diet/onion-diet.html

http://www.globalhealingcenter.com/nutrition/table-salt

http://wellnessmama.com/9166/sea-salt-spray-for-skin/

http://greatist.com/health/surprising-high-fiber-foods

http://blogs.scientificamerican.com/guest-blog/human-ancestors-were-nearly-all-vegetarians/

http://www.healthaliciousness.com/articles/foods-high-in-vitamin-B6.php

http://www.saywhatyouneedtosayblog.com/2012/11/05/slow-cooker-buffalo-chicken-chili/

http://www.everydayhealth.com/hs/thyroid-pictures/foods-to-eat/#02

Read more: http://www.care2.com/greenliving/health-benefits-of-epsom-salt-baths.html#ixzz3dE24L53V

http://chriskresser.com/selenium-the-missing-link-for-treating-hypothyroidism/

http://www.healthy-holistic-living.com/make-homemade-ketchup-just-2-minutes.html?t=DM

http://bembu.com/iodine-rich-foods

http://www.healthaliciousness.com/articles/zinc.php

http://www.whfoods.com/genpage.php/genpage.php?tname=nutrient&dbid=93

http://www.whfoods.com/genpage.php/genpage.php?tname=nutrient&dbid=83

National Institute of Health. Iodine. Office of Dietary Supplements. Fact Sheet for Health Professionals.

http://www.drfranklipman.com/which-is-the-safest-cookware/

http://www.livestrong.com/article/327754-how-many-calories-does-the-average-american-eat-daily/

http://fitlife.tv/10-amazing-benefits-of-pink-himalayan-salt/

http://nutritiondata.self.com/foods-00008700000000000000.html
(Foods highest in Tyrosine)

See more at: http://www.oxygenmag.com/article/is-tyrosine-an-all-purpose-chill-pill-8949#sthash.wUP5KTDL.dpuf

http://umm.edu/health/medical/altmed/supplement/tyrosine

Source: Tyrosine | University of Maryland Medical Center http://umm.edu/health/medical/altmed/supplement/tyrosine#ixzz3aCcHy6lp

http://lowthyroiddiet.com/foods-to-eat.htm

http://healthwyze.org/index.php/component/content/article/327-beware-of-deodorants-especially-the-safe-and-all-natural-ones.html

http://www.scientificamerican.com/article/bring-science-home-iodine-salt/

References' and my cited your sources of inspiration.

http://www.aucklandholisticcentre.co.nz/Holistic-Medicine-Holistic-Doctor-Auckland/sea-salt-himalayan-salt-and-a-short-word-on-iodine.html

http://ods.od.nih.gov/factsheets/Iodine-HealthProfessional/ National Institute of Health. Iodine. Office of Dietary Supplements. Fact Sheet for Health Professionals.

http://drhyman.com/blog/2010/05/20/a-7-step-plan-to-boost-your-low-thyroid-and-metabolis/#close

http://bembu.com/iodine-rich-foods

http://www.crunchybetty.com/battle-of-the-homemade-glass-cleaners

http://www.naturalnews.com/002693_personal_care_products_dryer_sheets.html

http://www.crunchybetty.com/getting-to-the-bottom-of-borax-is-it-safe-or-not

http://www.crunchybetty.com/nontoxic-homemade-oven-cleaner-will-it-work

http://foodbabe.com/2015/01/12/mexican-lentil-tortilla-soup/

http://bembu.com/iodine-rich-foods

http://thenakedlabel.com/blog/2013/01/17/whats-the-scoop-on-salt/

http://dailyhealthpost.com/3-reasons-to-love-himalayan-pink-salt/

http://www.globalhealingcenter.com/natural-health/iodine-foods/

http://www.santaclarasanjosechiropractor.com/index.php?p=149390

http://www.nationofchange.org/ultimate-paradox-us-over-fed-and-malnourished-nation-1372077901

http://www.aloeit.com/human-engine-our-bodies-health/

http://www.webmd.com/a-to-z-guides/hypothyroidism-topic-overview

http://www.mayoclinic.org/diseases-conditions/hypothyroidism/basics/symptoms/con-20021179

http://www.webmd.com/a-to-z-guides/hypothyroidism-topic-overview

http://hypothyroidmom.com/300-hypothyroidism-symptoms-yes-really/

http://www.womentowomen.com/thyroid-health/hypothyroid-symptoms-2/

http://www.medicinenet.com/hypothyroidism_symptoms/views.htm

http://www.medicalnewstoday.com/articles/163729.php

http://articles.mercola.com/sites/articles/archive/2011/08/13/fluoride-and-thyroid-dysfunction.aspx

http://thyroid.about.com/od/symptomsrisks/a/Why-Are-So-Many-People-Getting-Thyroid-Disease.htm

http://journaltimes.com/lifestyles/relationships-and-special-occasions/earthtalk-could-thyroid-problems-have-environmental-cause/article_91205880-50d4-11e0-a7bb-001cc4c002e0.html

http://www.rodalenews.com/2014-dirty-dozen

http://www.ewg.org/foodnews/

http://www.stopthethyroidmadness.com/long-and-pathetic/

http://www.livestrong.com/article/141120-the-dangers-epsom-salts/

http://thyroid.about.com/od/thyroiddrugtreatments/a/Coffee-Espresso-Thyroid-Medication-Levothyroxine.htm

http://www.ncbi.nlm.nih.gov/pmc/articles/PMC2293315/

http://articles.mercola.com/sites/articles/archive/2003/11/08/thyroid-health-part-two.aspx)

http://naturesnurtureblog.com/2011/06/01/how-to-naturally-freshen-your-laundry/

http://www.naturalnews.com/022902.html

http://www.livestrong.com/article/440180-what-are-benefits-of-not-eating-before-bed/)

http://www.redbookmag.com/body/healthy-eating/advice/g738/snacks-for-weight-loss/?slide=16 http://www.prevention.com/food/healthy-recipes/17-snacks-power-weight-loss?s=14

Serve with green salad. - See more at: http://www.hotzehwc.com/en-US/Resource-Center/Health-Wellness-Advice/July-2012/Vegetable-Quiche-Recipe.aspx#sthash.R7E2cDa2.dpuf

http://www.bellechevre.com/goat-cheese-is-sexy-skinny-smart/

http://www.foodnetwork.com/recipes/giada-de-laurentiis/goat-cheese-lentil-and-brown-rice-rolls-recipe2.html

http://articles.mercola.com/sites/articles/archive/2014/09/28/goat-cheese-benefits.aspx

http://www.womansday.com/recipefinder/chickpea-red-pepper-soup-quinoa-recipe-wdy0214

http://www.huffingtonpost.com/2013/08/06/facts-about-sweat_n_3709248.html

http://www.cheaprecipeblog.com/2013/01/the-10-food-day-tomato-and-lentil-soup-recipe/

http://www.ncbi.nlm.nih.gov/pubmed/21896934

http://jn.nutrition.org/content/137/4/1087.long

http://www.ncbi.nlm.nih.gov/pubmed/22211512

http://www.ncbi.nlm.nih.gov/pubmed/20224659

http://www.food.com/recipe/lentil-and-quinoa-chili-507595

http://bembu.com/iodine-rich-foods

http://notyourstandard.com/date-and-fig-coconut-rolls/

1. Mazokopakis EE, Starakis IK, Papadomanolaki MG, Batistakis AG, Papadakis JA. Changes of bone mineral density in pre-menopausal women with differentiated thyroid cancer receiving L-thyroxine suppressive therapy. Curr Med Res Opin. 2006;22:1369–73. [PubMed]

2. Mandel SJ, Brent GA, Larsen PR. Levothyroxine therapy in patients with thyroid disease. Ann Intern Med. 1993;119:492–502. [PubMed]

3. Singh N, Singh PN, Hershman JM. Effect of calcium carbonate on the absorption of levothyroxine . JAMA. 2000;283:2822–5. [PubMed]

4. Singh N, Weisler SL, Hershman JM. The acute effect of calcium carbonate on the intestinal absorption of levothyroxine. Thyroid. 2001; 11:967–71. [PubMed]

5. Neafsey PJ. Levothyroxine and calcium interaction: timing is everything. Home Health Nurse. 2004; 22:338–9. [PubMed]
6. Mazokopakis EE. Counseling patients receiving levothyroxine (L-T4) and calcium carbonate. Mil Med. 2006;171:vii,1094. [PubMed]

[No authors listed]. Iodine. Monograph. Altern Med Rev 2010; 15(3):273–278.

Leung AM and Braverman LE. Iodine-induced thyroid dysfunction. Curr Opin Endocrinol Diabetes Obes 2012; 19(5): 414–419.

Brahmbhatt SR et al. Thyroid ultrasound is the best prevalence indicator for assessment of iodine deficiency disorders: a study in rural/tribal schoolchildren from Gujarat (Western India). European Journal of Endocrinology 2000;143:37–46.

Brahmbhatt SR et al. Study of biochemical prevalence indicators for the assessment of iodine deficiency disorders in adults at field conditions in Gujarat (India). Asia Pacific J Clin Nutr 2001; 10(1):51–57.

http://www.mayoclinic.org/diseases-conditions/hypothyroidism/expert-answers/hypothyroidism/faq-20058536

http://www.myrecipes.com/recipe/tuna-white-bean-salad-2

http://www.eatingwell.com/recipes/sardine_greek_salad.html

http://www.everydayhealth.com/health-report/thyroid-pictures/foods-to-eat.aspx#/slide-2

http://www.abouthypothyroidism.net/some-breakfast-options-that-help-to-manage-hypothyroidism-better-than-ever

http://products.mercola.com/coconut-flour/

http://authoritynutrition.com/15-low-carb-bread-recipes/

http://www.cutthewheat.com/2013/05/cheesy-garlic-bread-grain-and-gluten.html

http://mariamindbodyhealth.com/baby-corn-bread-2/

http://www.thrive-style.com/2012/02/fancy-grilled-cheese-on-coconut-flour-flatbread-gluten-and-grain-free/

http://www.thrive-style.com/2012/04/coconut-flour-flatbread-grilled-cheese-recipe-update-pizza-flavor/

http://cavemanketo.com/faux-bread-quest-holy-grail-almond-buns/

http://divaliciousrecipesinthecity.com/2011/10/14/healthy-gluten-free-and-low-carb-bread/

http://smittenkitchen.com/blog/2013/03/coconut-bread/

http://www.wholefoodsmarket.com/recipe/coconut-bread

http://www.myrecipes.com/recipe/coconut-banana-bread-with-lime-glaze-10000001654705/

http://deliciouslyorganic.net/coffee-cake-coconut-flour-recipe-gluten-free/

http://www.libbylouer.com/cranberry-orange-coconut-flour-bread/

http://www.amazingpaleo.com/2012/08/15/simple-coconut-bread/

http://www.food.com/recipe/ka-zucchini-coconut-quick-bread-478123

http://thyroid.about.com/cs/shames/a/fluoride.htm

http://thyroid.about.com/od/thyroidbasicsthyroid101/ss/preventthyroid_7.htm

http://foodmatters.tv/articles-1/cheers-to-drinking-warm-lemon-water

http://www.lifehack.org/articles/lifestyle/11-benefits-lemon-water-you-didnt-know-about.html

http://www.buzzle.com/articles/breakfast-options-for-hypothyroid-patients.html

http://www.buzzle.com/articles/breakfast-options-for-hypothyroid-patients.html

http://bluewhitekitchen.blogspot.com/2011/06/diet-for-hypothyroidism.html

http://www.webmd.com/food-recipes/guide/are-you-getting-enough-vitamin-d

http://ods.od.nih.gov/factsheets/VitaminD-HealthProfessional/

http://health.howstuffworks.com/wellness/food-nutrition/vitamin-supplements/how-much-vitamin-d-from-sun1.htm

http://www.naturalendocrinesolutions.com/articles/personal-thyroid-diet/

http://www.livestrong.com/article/440180-what-are-benefits-of-not-eating-before-bed/

*Eating before bed slows metabolism and encourages weight gain, says Dr. Mark Hyman in his book *Ultrametabolism*.

*The National Institutes of Health's Digestive Diseases Information Clearinghouse recommends not eating two to three hours before bed to help control the symptoms of GERD.

*Eating at night might upset your body's natural day/night cycle and lead to poor-quality sleep, says Erika Gebel, writing for "Diabetes Forecast."

*According to Columbia University Health Services. Calories you consume late at night have the same energy value as calories you consume at any other time.

http://articles.mercola.com/sites/articles/archive/2003/11/08/thyroid-health-part-two.aspx

http://wellnessmama.com/36/thyroid-problems-coconut-oil/

http://healthimpactnews.com/2013/get-off-your-thyroid-medication-and-start-consuming-coconut-oil/

http://www.ncbi.nlm.nih.gov/pubmed/11880549/

http://www.doctoroz.com/videos/surprising-health-benefits-coconut-oil

http://innersourcehealth.com/

Pina LoGiudice ND, LAc, Siobhan Bleakney, ND, and Peter Bongiorno ND, LAc Co-Medical Directors of Inner Source Health in New York

http://www.freecoconutrecipes.com/index.cfm/2011/8/29/skillet-glazed-corn-with-ginger-lime-and-coconut

http://alldayidreamaboutfood.com/2011/12/almond-flour-bread-and-french-toast-low-carb-and-gluten-free.html#0sv5s6 CudFCjKPEG.99

http://www.agirlworthsaving.net/2013/03/paleo-pretzels.html

http://gourmandeinthekitchen.com/2012/crisp-rosemary-parmesan-flatbread-with-arugula-recipe/

http://www.averiecooks.com/2014/02/cinnamon-spice-apple-sauce-bread-with-honey-butter.html

http://www.sunstreakedandstyled.com/2013/02/paleo-blueberry-coconut-cups.html

http://products.mercola.com/himalayan-salt/

http://www.myrecipes.com/recipe/curried-chickpea-stew-50400 000109633/

http://www.macheesmo.com/2010/04/chickpea-patties/

http://allrecipes.com/recipe/easy-garam-masala/

http://www.skinnytaste.com/2014/04/quinoa-chickpea-and-avocado-salad.html

http://www.womansday.com/recipefinder/chickpea-red-pepper-soup-quinoa-recipe-wdy0214

http://www.santaclarasanjosechiropractor.com/index.php?p=149390

http://www.nationofchange.org/ultimate-paradox-us-overfed-and-malnourished-nation-1372077901

http://www.aloeit.com/human-engine-our-bodies-health/

http://www.webmd.com/a-to-z-guides/hypothyroidism-topic-overview

http://www.mayoclinic.org/diseases-conditions/hypothyroidism/basics/symptoms/con-20021179

http://www.webmd.com/a-to-z-guides/hypothyroidism-topic-overview

http://hypothyroidmom.com/300-hypothyroidism-symptoms-yes-really/

http://www.womentowomen.com/thyroid-health/hypothyroid-symptoms-2/

http://www.medicinenet.com/hypothyroidism_symptoms/views.htm

http://www.stopthethyroidmadness.com/long-and-pathetic/

http://www.instructables.com/id/Microwave-Popcorn%3A-Home-made,-cheap-and-easy/

http://www.snack-girl.com/snack/healthy-apple-crisp/

http://www.snack-girl.com/snack/fig-chocolate-recipe/

http://www.snack-girl.com/snack/easy-black-bean-soup/

http://www.fastcoexist.com/1677855/6-steps-to-avoiding-bpa-in-your-daily-life

http://www.seattleorganicrestaurants.com/vegan-whole-foods/avoid-canned-food/

http://www.seattleorganicrestaurants.com/vegan-whole-foods/avoid-canned-food/

http://www.yummly.com/recipe/Pink-a-colada-367288?columns=6&position=7%2F58

http://www.yummly.com/recipe/external/Coconut-creamsicle-margaritas-357629

http://www.yummly.com/recipe/external/Pineapple-Coconut-Sour-484926

http://www.yummly.com/recipe/external/Pumpkin-Martini-637646

http://www.huffingtonpost.ca/diana-herrington/7-benefits-of-quinoa_b_3363619.html

http://www.bbcgoodfood.com/howto/guide/health-benefits-quinoa

http://www.bbcgoodfood.com/recipes/2364643/spicy-tuna-quinoa-salad

http://www.realsimple.com/food-recipes/browse-all-recipes/zucchini-quinoa-stuffing

http://www.medicalnewstoday.com/articles/280244.php

http://www.simplyrecipes.com

http://www.motherearthliving.com/cooking-methods/smart-foods-for-hypothyroidism.aspx#ixzz3MFgVKwB2

http://thesimpleveganista.blogspot.com/2012/11/roasted-butter-nut-squash-soup.html

http://pumpsandiron.com/2014/02/11/apple-banana-quinoa-breakfast-cups/

http://www.thespiffycookie.com/2013/02/20/cinnamon-apple-quinoa-parfaits/

http://preventionrd.com/2012/03/cinnamon-apple-quinoa-parfait/

http://www.motherearthliving.com/cooking-methods/smart-foods-for-hypothyroidism.aspx#ixzz3MFdyDXAR

http://whatsfordinner-momwhatsfordinner.blogspot.com/2013/03/poached-eggs-over-cauliflower-quinoa.html

http://www.mercola.com/Downloads/bonus/dangers-of-non-stick-cookware/report.aspx

Takahashi Y, Kipnis DM, Daughaday WH Growth hormone secretion during sleep. J Clin Invest 1968;47:2079–2090.

Weitzman E. D., Fukushima D, Nogeire C, Roffwarg H, Gallagher T. F., Hellman L. Twenty-four hour pattern of the episodic secretion of cortisol in normal subjects. J Clin Endocriol Metab 1971;33:14–22.

Flegal, K. M. et al. Prevalence and Trends in Obesity Among US Adults, 1999–2008 JAMA. 2010;303(3):235–241.

Interviews with Melanie Polk, registered dietitian and director of nutrition education for the American Institute of Cancer Research

Interview with Marion Nestle, Marion Nestle, PhD, MPH, Chair of the Department of Nutrition and Food Studies at New York University

Interview with Barbara Gollman, registered dietitian and spokesperson for the American Dietetic Association

Nestle, M. and M. F. Jacobson. Halting the obesity epidemic: A public health policy approach. Public Health Reports, January/February 2000. 115:12–24.

The American Institute for Cancer Research. The New American Plate: A timely approach to eating for healthy life and healthy weight.

Fung, T. T. et al. Association between dietary patterns and plasma biomarkers of obesity and cardiovascular disease risk. American Journal of Clinical Nutrition, January 2001. 73:61–67.

Centers for Disease Control. Overweight. April 2006. http://www.cdc.gov/nchs/fastats/overwt.htm

Alliance for a Healthier Generation. Alliance for a Healthier Generation Clinton Foundation and American Heart Association and Industry Leaders Set Healthy School Beverage Guidelines for US Schools. May 2006.

US Department of Agriculture. How much food from the meat and bans group is needed daily? http://www.mypyramid.gov/pyramid/meat_amount.aspx

Ogden, CL et al. High Body Mass Index for Age Among US Children and Adolescents, 2003-2006. Journal of the American Medical Association. 299(20):2401-2405. May 2008. http://jama.ama-assn.org/cgi/content/short/299/20/2401

Higdon J, Delage B, Williams D, et al: Cruciferous vegetables and human cancer risk: epidemiologic evidence and mechanistic basis. Pharmacol Res 2007;55:224–236.

Wu QJ, Yang Y, Vogtmann E, et al: Cruciferous vegetables intake and the risk of colorectal cancer: a meta-analysis of observational studies. Ann Oncol 2012.

Liu X, Lv K: Cruciferous vegetables intake is inversely associated with risk of breast cancer: A meta-analysis. Breast 2012.

Liu B, Mao Q, Lin Y, et al: The association of cruciferous vegetables intake and risk of bladder cancer: a meta-analysis. World J Urol 2012.

Liu B, Mao Q, Cao M, et al: Cruciferous vegetables intake and risk of prostate cancer: a meta-analysis. Int J Urol 2012;19:134–141.

Lam TK, Gallicchio L, Lindsley K, et al: Cruciferous vegetable consumption and lung cancer risk: a systematic review. Cancer Epidemiol Biomarkers Prev 2009;18:184–195.

Bosetti C, Negri E, Kolonel L, et al: A pooled analysis of case-control studies of thyroid cancer. VII. Cruciferous and other vegetables (International). Cancer Causes Control 2002;13:765–775.

Dal Maso L, Bosetti C, La Vecchia C, et al: Risk factors for thyroid cancer: an epidemiological review focused on nutritional factors. Cancer Causes Control 2009;20:75–86.

Phytochemicals and Other Dietary Factors 2nd edition: Thieme; 2013

Krajcovicova-Kudlackova M, Buckova K, Klimes I, et al: Iodine deficiency in vegetarians and vegans. Ann Nutr Metab 2003; 47:183–185.

Leung AM, Lamar A, He X, et al: Iodine status and thyroid function of Boston-area vegetarians and vegans. J Clin Endocrinol Metab 2011;96:E1303–1307.

Office of Dietary Supplements, National Institutes of Health. Dietary Supplement Fact Sheet: Iodine.

Tonstad S, Nathan E, Oda K, et al: Vegan diets and hypothyroidism. Nutrients 2013;5:4642–4652.

McMillan M, Spinks EA, Fenwick GR: Preliminary observations on the effect of dietary brussels sprouts on thyroid function. Hum Toxicol 1986;5:15–19.

Chu M, Seltzer TF: Myxedema coma induced by ingestion of raw bok choy. N Engl J Med 2010;362:1945–1946.

Zhang X, Shu XO, Xiang YB, et al: Cruciferous vegetable consumption is associated with a reduced risk of total and cardiovascular disease mortality. Am J Clin Nutr 2011;94:240–246.

Fenwick GR, Heaney RK, Mullin WJ. Glucosinolates and their breakdown products in food and food plants. Crit Rev Food Sci Nutr. 1983;18(2):123–201

Chu M, Seltzer TF. Myxedema coma induced by ingestion of raw bok choy. N Engl J Med. 2010;362(20):1945–1946.

Online places to visit:

Flouridealert.org
https://donatenow.networkforgood.org/1415005
http://www.mercola.com/Downloads/bonus/dangers-of-nonstick-cookware/report.aspx

Recipes (as in the measured list of ingredients) *and* very short directions on how to combine those ingredients are not protected under the various forms of copyright law. This is because they fall under the designation of being the steps in a procedure and they're explicitly excluded from copyright.

Countries which are signatories to either the Berne convention or the Buenos Aires convention use the same basic standard to determine what is and isn't copyrighted although there are small local variations. However, the exclusion on procedures is not a local variation.

What *can* be copyrighted are the more complex directions that usually accompany the list of ingredients in modern recipes. As long as you rewrite any directions to be in your own words you've followed the law. Cooking something from a recipe recorded by someone else and selling it is legal.

ABOUT THE AUTHOR

A personal favorite quote of mine is "From stressed to blessed." I mean this, believe, and receive this. I've been battling hypothyroidism for years, and I wanted to create a user-friendly handbook to help anyone affected by this disorder. I've seen many doctors over the years and none offered me ideas on diet change. I've included recipes, ideas on solutions for a healthier home, what you should be eating and shouldn't, how to shed those extra pounds, regain your self-confidence and vitality back into your life. I want you to feel strong, sexy, and beautiful. This is my heartfelt guide to you. Together, once again, you can start to gain that wonderful life that you deserve. I am a student in this thing called *life*. I want to be remembered as a pioneer who thought, imagined, and inspired. What we feel at times is the impossible or unthinkable. Life is a wonderful journey. Laugh at yourself as much as possible! Never try to walk someone else's path. You are destined for your own path and journey. I can't be you, and you can't be me. It's up to you to accept your journey and walk your path in life. Let's kick hypothyroidism's booty together!

CPSIA information can be obtained at www.ICGtesting.com
Printed in the USA
BVOW05s1227230416

445248BV00001B/3/P

9 781682 893685